Paleo Diet

30 Day Paleo Challenge to Lose 22 Pounds with 120 Mouth-Watering Paleo Recipes

Table of Contents

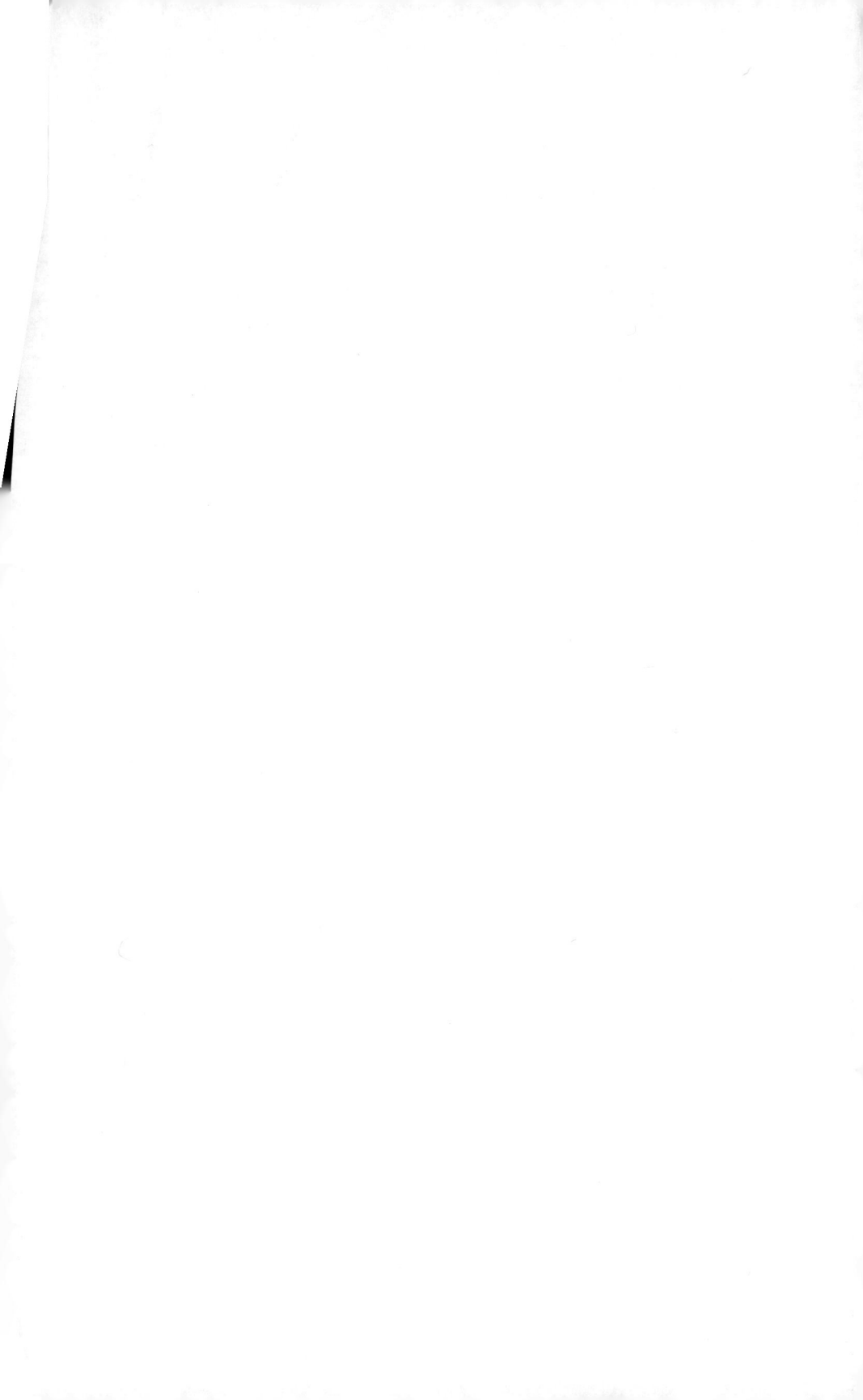

Introduction

I want to thank you and congratulate you for purchasing the book, *"Paleo Diet: 120 Paleo Recipes for Everyday Cooks ".*

This book contains proven steps and strategies on how to make 120 paleo recipes that won't break the bank or your waistline.

The Paleo Diet is more than just a diet. It's living the lifestyle of our not so distant ancestors, who were free from cancers, cardiovascular disease, and many other modern-day diseases caused by a diet high in processed foods and fast food. You'll rediscover the delicious taste of fresh foods when you cook with the recipes in this book.

Thanks again for purchasing this book, I hope you enjoy it!

Breakfast

Hash Brown and Sausage Breakfast Casserole
Serves: 4

Ingredients

- 8 Eggs
- 2 Sausages, Sliced And Cooked
- ½ C. Coconut Milk
- 2 Sweet Potatoes, Shredded
- 1 Red Onion, Chopped
- 2 Cloves of garlic, Finely Chopped
- 1 Tbsp. Fresh Basil, Finely Chopped
- 1 Tbsp. Fresh Chives, Finely Chopped
- 2 Tbsp. Cooking Fat
- Salt And Pepper

Directions

1. Preheat your oven to 350 degrees.
2. Melt cooking fat in a skillet over medium heat.
3. Sauté the garlic and onion for five minutes.
4. Add the sweet potatoes and sauté for eight minutes. Remove from the heat and put into a casserole dish.

5. Whisk the egg, chives, milk, and basil together in a bowl. Season to taste with salt and pepper.
6. Pour the egg mix over the sweet potatoes and top with the sausage pieces.
7. Bake for half an hour.
8. Allow it to rest five minutes before serving.

Breakfast Scramble with Sweet Potatoes
Serves: 4

Ingredients

- 2 C. Sweet Potatoes, Chopped
- 8 Eggs
- ¼ C. Almond Milk
- 1 Green Onion, Thinly Sliced
- 2 Tsp. Chili Powder
- 2 Tsp. Dried Oregano
- ½ C. Fresh Salsa
- 2 Tbsp. Ghee
- Salt And Pepper

Directions

1. Bring the water to a boil in a pot and add the sweet potatoes, cook for ten minutes. Drain the water, season the potatoes to taste, and set them aside.
2. Whisk the eggs, chili powder, milk, and oregano together in a bowl. Season to taste.
3. Melt the ghee in another skillet over high heat.
4. Pour the egg into the skillet and cook until the egg has set.
5. Serve the scrambled eggs with the sweet potatoes, salsa, and green onion slices.

Bacon and Jalapeno Egg Cups
Serves: 4

Ingredients
- 10 Eggs
- 12 Bacon Slices, Par-Cooked
- ½ Onion, Chopped
- 4 Jalapeno Peppers, Sliced And Seeds Removed
- ¼ C. Almond Milk
- ½ C. Bell Pepper, Chopped
- ½ Tsp. Garlic Powder
- Salt And Pepper

Directions
1. Preheat the oven to 375 degrees.
2. In a bowl, add the milk, eggs, and garlic powder and season to taste. Whisk until it's combined.
3. Take out a muffin tin and line the cups with a slice of bacon.
4. Fill the tins with the egg mix and top with the remaining ingredients.
5. Bake for twenty minutes.

Tomato Sauce Eggs

Serves: 4

Ingredients

- 6 Eggs
- 8 Slices Of Bacon, Diced And Cooked
- 1 Onion, Roughly Chopped
- 3 Cloves Of Garlic, Finely Chopped
- 1 Tbsp. Chili Powder
- ½ C. Chicken Stock
- 28 Oz. Tomatoes, Chopped
- 2 Potatoes, Chopped
- Cooking Fat
- Salt And Pepper

Directions

1. Melt the fat in a skillet over high heat and sauté the onion until it's soft.
2. Add the garlic and sauté another minute.
3. Pour the stock in and scrape up the onion bits. Add the tomatoes.
4. Season with chili powder and the salt and pepper and simmer for fifteen minutes.
5. Transfer to a blender and puree until it's smooth.
6. Melt more cooking fat into the skillet.
7. Sauté the potatoes for a few minutes or until they're browned.
8. Pour the sauce over the potatoes and simmer twelve minutes.

9. Crack the eggs into the sauce.
10. Sprinkle with the crumbled bacon and cook for ten minutes, covered.

Spinach, Sweet Potato, and Bacon Quiche
Serves: 4

Ingredients

- 5 Eggs, Beaten
- 4 Sweet Potatoes, Peeled And Sliced
- 2 C. Fresh Spinach
- 3 Bacon Pieces, Cooked And Crumbled
- 1 Onion, Sliced
- 1 Clove Of Garlic, Finely Chopped
- 2 Tbsp. Fresh Chives
- 2 Tsp. Olive Oil
- Cooking Fat
- Salt And Pepper

Directions

1. Preheat your oven to 400 degrees.
2. Put the potato slice sin a pie dish in a circular pattern to make a crust.
3. Drizzle the potatoes with the oil and season to taste.
4. Bake for twenty minutes.
5. Melt some fat in a skillet over medium heat and sauté the onion and garlic.
6. Add the spinach and sauté until it's wilted, two to three minutes. Set it aside to cool.
7. Once the potatoes are finished, lower the oven temperature to 375 degrees.
8. Combine the eggs with the spinach, chives, and bacon.

9. Pour this over the sweet potato crust.
10. Bake for thirty-five minutes.

Sausage and Eggs Breakfast Hash
Serves: 4

Ingredients

- 8 Eggs
- 2 Sweet Potatoes, Chopped
- 4 Sausages, Casing Removed
- 1 Bell Pepper, Chopped
- 1 Onion, Chopped
- Green Onions, Sliced
- 1 Tsp. Chili Powder
- ½ Tsp. Garlic Powder
- ½ Tsp. Dried Oregano
- 1 Tbsp. Olive Oil
- Cooking Fat
- Salt And Pepper

Directions

1. Preheat the oven to 400 degrees.
2. Put the sweet potato cubes into a bowl and drizzle them with the oil, season with the chili powder, garlic, and oregano, and season with salt and pepper to taste.
3. Spread them onto a baking sheet in a single layer. Bake for half an hour.
4. Melt the cooking fat in a skillet over medium heat.
5. Sauté the onions and peppers for three minutes.

6. Add the sausages to the pan and cook until it's browned, around six minutes. Add the sweet potatoes and stir it all together.
7. Remove the mix from the pan. Add more cooking fat and cook the eggs.
8. Divide the potato sausage mix amongst the plates and top each one with a fried egg.
9. Garnish with the green onions.

Scrambled Eggs with Apples and Onions
Serves: 4

Ingredients
- 8 Eggs, Beaten
- ½ Red Onion, Chopped
- 1 Granny Smith Apple, Chopped
- 1 Celery Rib, Chopped
- Fresh Chives, Finely Chopped
- Cooking Fat
- Salt And Pepper

Directions
1. Melt the fat in a skillet over medium heat.
2. Sauté the onion and celery for three minutes.
3. Sauté the onion for two minutes.
4. Pour the beaten eggs into the apple mix and stir slowly until the eggs are almost done.
5. Remove it from the heat, season to taste, and allow it to rest for two minutes.
6. Serve garnished with chives.

Spinach and Smoked Salmon Baked Eggs

Serves: 4

Ingredients

- 1 Smoked Salmon Fillet, Cut Into Chunks
- 2 Shallots, Sliced
- 4 Eggs
- 10 Oz. Baby Spinach
- Fresh Chives, Finely Chopped
- 4 Tbsp. Coconut Milk
- Cooking Fat
- Salt And Pepper

Directions

1. Preheat the oven to 350 degrees.
2. Preheat a skillet to medium and melt the fat.
3. Sauté the shallots for four minutes.
4. Wilt the spinach in the pan.
5. Pour the milk into the pan and season to taste. Cook another minute.
6. Divide the spinach amongst four oven safe dishes.
7. Make a well in each one and crack an egg into it.
8. Divide the salmon pieces amongst the dishes.
9. Bake for twelve to fifteen minutes.
10. Garnish with chives and serve.

Sweet Potato Nest Eggs
Serves: 4-6

Ingredients
- 12 Eggs
- 4 Sweet Potatoes
- 6 Slices Of Bacon, Cooked And Crumbled
- Cooking Fat, Melted
- 2 Tbsp. Fresh Chives, Finely Chopped
- Salt And Pepper

Directions
1. Preheat the oven to 400 degrees.
2. Bake the potatoes forty minutes.
3. Let the potatoes cool down and peel them. Grate them into a bowl and season them to taste.
4. Grease a muffin tin liberally with fat.
5. Scoop three tablespoons of sweet potato into the muffin cups. Press down with your fingers to make a nest shape.
6. Return the shells to the oven and bake ten minutes.
7. Crack and egg into each next and season to taste. Sprinkle with fresh chives.
8. Bake twelve minutes.
9. Remove the nests from the pan and serve with crumbled bacon.

Smoked Salmon Scrambled Eggs

Serves: 2

Ingredients

- 4 Eggs
- 2 Tbsp. Coconut Milk
- 4 Slices Smoked Salmon, Chopped
- Fresh Chives, Finely Chopped
- Cooking Fat
- Salt And Pepper

Directions

1. Whisk the eggs, milk, and chives together. Season to taste.
2. Melt some cooking fat in the skillet and add the eggs.
3. Scramble the eggs as you cook.
4. When the eggs begin to set, add the salmon and cook for two minutes.
5. Serve garnished with chives.

Red Meats

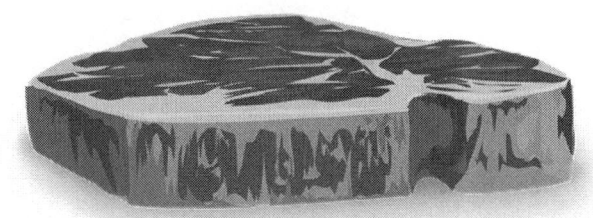

Greek Meatballs
Serves: 4

Ingredients
- 1 ½ Lbs. Ground Beef Or Lamb
- 1 Egg, Beaten
- ¼ C. Fresh Parsley. Finely Chopped
- 2 Cloves Of Garlic, Finely Chopped
- 2 Tbsp. Tomato Paste
- 1 Tsp. Dried Mint
- 1 Tbsp. Dried Oregano
- Salt And Pepper

Directions
1. Preheat the oven to 350 degrees.
2. In a bowl, add the ground meat, parsley, egg, tomato paste, garlic, mint, and oregano. Season to taste.
3. Mix it together and make meatballs.
4. Put them on a baking sheet and cook in the oven for twenty-five minutes.

Burgers
Serves: 4

Ingredients
- 1 Lb. Ground Beef
- 8 Bacon Strips, Cooked
- 8 Portobello Mushrooms, Stem Removed
- 1 Egg
- 4 Onion Slices
- 4 Tomato Slices
- Fresh Lettuce
- 2 Tbsp. Olive Oil
- Salt And Pepper

Directions
1. Preheat the grill to medium.
2. Combine the beef and egg in a bowl and season to taste.
3. Shape the beef into four patties.
4. Rub the mushrooms with oil and season to taste.
5. Grill the burgers seven minutes on either side, covered.
6. Grill the mushrooms six minutes on either side at the same time.
7. Serve the burger on the mushrooms topped with the bacon, onion, tomato, and lettuce.

Zucchini Boats with Steak

Serves: 4

Ingredients

- 4 Zucchini, Sliced In Half Lengthwise
- 1 Large Yellow Onion, Sliced
- 1 Lb. Thinly Sliced Roast Beef, Diced Small
- 6 Oz. Button Mushrooms, Sliced
- 2 Cloves Of Garlic, Finely Chopped
- 1 Bell Pepper, Chopped
- 1 Tbsp. Olive Oil
- Cooking Fat
- Salt And Pepper

Directions

1. Preheat the oven to 400 degrees.
2. Scoop the zucchini out to make a boat with a hollow center.
3. Brush them with oil and season to taste.
4. Bake in the oven for twenty minutes.
5. Melt fat in a skillet and put it over medium heat.
6. Sauté the onion and garlic for three minutes.
7. Sauté the bell pepper and mushrooms for five minutes.
8. Add the beef and season it all to taste. Cook for three minutes, stirring.

9. Fill the zucchini slices with the skillet mix and serve.

Zucchini and Veal Rolls
Serves: 4

Ingredients
- 8 Veal Scallops
- ¼ C. Balsamic Vinegar
- 2 Zucchini, Quartered
- 2 Tsp. Garlic Powder
- 2 Tbsp. Olive Oil
- Salt And Pepper

Directions
1. Preheat the grill to medium.
2. Use a meat mallet to flatten the veal.
3. Season with salt and pepper.
4. Season the zucchini with the salt, pepper, and garlic powder.
5. Grill the zucchini in either side for two minutes.
6. Remove it from the grill.
7. Roll the veal around the zucchini quarters.
8. Combine the oil and balsamic vinegar in a bowl.
9. Brush the rolls with the vinegar mix and grill for three minutes on either side.

Butternut Squash Lasagna
Serves: 4

Ingredients
- 1.5 Lbs. Ground Beef
- 1 Large Butternut Squash, Thinly Sliced
- 4 C. Tomato Sauce
- 4 Oz. Tomato Paste
- 3 Cloves Of Garlic, Finely Chopped
- 1 Onion, Finely Chopped
- 1 Tsp. Dried Oregano
- 1 Tsp. Dried Basil
- Cooking Fat
- Salt And Pepper

Directions
1. Preheat the oven to 400 degrees.
2. Melt the fat and sauté the onion and garlic five minutes.
3. Add the beef and cook six minutes.
4. Add the sauce, paste, oregano, basil, and season it all with salt and pepper. Turn the heat down and simmer ten minutes.
5. In a baking dish, alternate the squash slices with meat sauce. Keep making layers until you use all the ingredients.
6. Bake twenty-five minutes.

Beef Sirloin with Herb Marinade
Serves: 4

Ingredients
- (2) 15-Oz. Beef Sirloin Steaks
- Salt And Pepper
- 1 C. Extra Virgin Olive Oil
- 3 Cloves Of Garlic, Finely Chopped
- 2 Shallots, Finely Chopped
- 2 Tbsp. Fresh Parsley, Finely Chopped
- 3 Tbsp. Fresh Basil, Finely Chopped
- 2 Tbsp. Fresh Rosemary, Roughly Chopped
- 2 Tsp. Dried Oregano
- 2 Tbsp. Fresh Thyme, Roughly Chopped
- 3 Tbsp. Red Wine Vinegar
- Salt And Pepper

Directions
1. In a bowl, combine the oil through the salt and pepper.
2. Pour half the marinade into a container and add the steaks. Marinade for twenty minutes at room temperature.
3. Preheat a grill.
4. Cook the steaks seven minutes on either side.
5. Spread the marinade over a cutting board and press both sides of the steaks into it.

6. Slice the steaks and serve.

Beef, Ginger, and Mushroom Stir-Fry
Serves: 4

Ingredients
- 1 Lb. Sirloin, Cut Into Thin Strips
- 2 Cloves Of Garlic, Finely Chopped
- 4 Oz. Shiitake Mushrooms, Halved
- 8 Oz. Cremini Mushrooms, Sliced
- 3 C. Kale, Chopped
- Cooking Fat
- ¾ C. Beef Stock
- 3 Tbsp. Rice Wine Vinegar
- 1 Garlic Clove, Finely Chopped
- 1 Inch Ginger, Finely Chopped
- Salt And Pepper

Directions
1. Add the beef stock through the salt and pepper to a bowl and whisk.
2. Add the steak to the marinade and toss to coat. Refrigerate for fifteen minutes.
3. Heat the fat in a skillet over high heat.
4. Remove the steak from the marinade and reserve the marinade.
5. Add the garlic and steak to the pan and sauté for four minutes.
6. Remove the steak and set it aside.
7. Add the kale, mushrooms, and reserved marinade and cook another four minutes.

8. Return the steak to the skillet and stir to combine.
9. Serve.

Korean Short Ribs
Serves: 4

Ingredients
- 4 Lbs. Beef Short Ribs
- ½ C. Raw Honey
- ½ C. Coconut Aminos
- ½ C. Water
- ¼ C. White Wine Vinegar
- 1 Asian Pear, Peeled And Finely Grated
- 2 Green Onions, Thinly Sliced
- 4 Tbsp. Garlic, Finely Chopped
- Pepper

Directions
1. Make the sauce by combining everything but the ribs in a bowl. Season to taste.
2. Put the ribs in a plastic bag and cover with the sauce. Refrigerate for four hours.
3. Preheat the oven to 300 degrees.
4. Put the ribs in a Dutch oven with the marinade.
5. Roast until cooked through, two hours.
6. Transfer to a serving platter and serve.

Ground Beef Tacos

Serves: 4

Ingredients

- 2 Lbs. Ground Beef
- 1 Green Bell Pepper, Chopped
- 1 Tomato, Chopped
- 1 Onion, Chopped
- 1 C. Shredded Lettuce
- Homemade Salsa
- Toppings
- Fresh Cilantro, For Garnishing
- 1 Tbsp. Chili Powder
- ½ Tsp. Paprika
- 1 Tsp. Ground Cumin
- ½ Tsp. Garlic Powder
- ½ Tsp. Dried Oregano
- Salt And Pepper

Directions

1. Brown the ground beef and onion for ten minutes.
2. Combine the chili powder through the salt and pepper in a bowl.
3. Stir the seasoning into the meat. Reduce the heat to low and let it simmer ten minutes.

4. Layer the beef mix, lettuce, tomatoes, and bell pepper, along with any other toppings, into the taco shells.
5. Serve with salsa.

Mexican Steak with Mushrooms

Serves: 4

Ingredients

- 1.5 Lbs. Flank Steak
- 1 Onion, Thinly Sliced
- 2 Bell Peppers, Sliced
- 3 Cloves Garlic
- 8 Oz. Mushrooms, Quartered
- ¼ Tsp. Chili Powder
- ¼ Tsp. Cumin
- 1 Avocado, Sliced
- Cooking Fat
- Salt And Pepper
- ¼ C. Olive Oil
- 4 Cloves Garlic, Finely Chopped
- 3 Tbsp. Lime Juice
- 1 Tsp. Chili Powder
- 1 Tsp. Cumin
- Salt And Pepper

Directions

1. Combine the olive oil through the salt and pepper together in a plastic bag.
2. Add the steak and toss with the marinade. Refrigerate fifteen minutes to two hours.
3. Preheat the grill to medium heat.
4. Remove the steak from the marinade.

5. Grill the steak on either side for six minutes.
6. Transfer the steak to a cutting board and allow it to rest ten minutes.
7. Melt some fat in a skillet over high heat.
8. Add the bell peppers, onions, and garlic and sauté five minutes.
9. Add the mushrooms and sauté another two minutes.
10. Add the chili powder and cumin and season to taste. Cook for two minutes and remove it from the heat.
11. Slice the steak into strips and serve with the vegetables and avocado slices.

Balsamic Steak Rolls

Serves: 4

Ingredients

- 2 Lb. Skirt Steak, Sliced
- 1 Bell Pepper, Sliced
- 1 Carrot, Sliced
- 5 Green Onions, Sliced
- ½ Zucchini, Sliced
- 2 Cloves Of Garlic, Finely Chopped
- ½ Tsp. Dried Basil
- ½ Tsp. Dried Oregano
- Cooking Fat
- Salt And Pepper
- 1 Tbsp. Ghee
- ¼ C. Balsamic Vinegar
- 2 Tbsp. Shallots, Finely Chopped
- 1 Tbsp. Honey
- ¼ C. Beef Stock
- Salt And Pepper

Directions

1. Season the steak with salt and pepper and set them aside.
2. Melt the ghee in a skillet over medium heat.
3. Sauté the shallots for three minutes.
4. Add the honey, vinegar, beef stock, and season again.

5. Bring it to a boil, then a simmer, and cook until the liquid has reduced to half. Put in a bowl.
6. In the skillet, add more fat and sauté the garlic two minutes. Add the rest of the vegetables and cook for four minutes.
7. Season with basil, oregano, and more salt and pepper. Put in another bowl.
8. Arrange a pile of vegetables on the center of every beef slice. Tightly roll the meat around it and secure with a toothpick.
9. Return the rolls to the skillet and cook over high heat on all sides until the meat is done.
10. Remove the toothpicks and spoon the sauce over the rolls. Serve.

Poultry

Spinach and Artichoke Chicken
Serves: 4

Ingredients
- 6 Chicken Thighs
- 14 Oz. Artichokes, Drained
- 1 Red Onion, Sliced
- 6 Oz. Baby Spinach
- 1 Yellow Onion, Sliced
- 2 Cloves Of Garlic, Chopped
- 2 Carrots, Sliced
- 1 C. Chicken Stock
- Cooking Fat
- Salt And Pepper

Directions
1. Preheat the oven to 425 degrees.
2. Season the chicken with salt and pepper.
3. Melt the fat in a Dutch oven over high heat.
4. Add the chicken and brown for five minutes on either side.
5. Remove from the skillet and set it aside.
6. Add the onions, artichokes, and carrots to the skillet.
7. Cook until the vegetables are tender.

8. Add the spinach and garlic and sauté another minute.
9. Return the chicken and pour in the stock.
10. Put it in the oven and bake for twenty minutes.
11. Remove from the oven and allow to rest five minutes before serving.

Cajun Chicken with Mushrooms

Serves: 4

Ingredients

- 6 Oz. Mushrooms, Sliced
- 4 Chicken Breasts, Cut Into Chunks
- 1 ½ C. Onions, Chopped
- 1 ½ C. Celery, Chopped
- 1 C. Chopped Green Bell Peppers
- ½ C. Red Bell Peppers
- 2 Cloves Of Garlic, Finely Chopped
- 2 C. Chicken Stock
- ½ Tsp. Cayenne Pepper
- 4 Drops Hot Sauce
- 2 Tbsp. Tapioca Starch
- ¼ C. Ghee
- Salt And Pepper

Directions

1. Preheat the skillet over medium heat and brown the chicken pieces on all sides.
2. Melt the ghee in a Dutch oven over medium heat.
3. Stir in the starch and keep stirring until its browned.
4. Add the celery, onions, peppers, and garlic and cook until it's just softened.
5. Pour in the stock and stir continuously.

6. Add the rest of the ingredients and season to taste.
7. Cover and simmer an hour.

Garlic Chicken

Serves: 4

Ingredients

- 4 Chicken Breasts
- ¼ C. Raw Honey
- ¼ C. Apple Cider Vinegar
- 2 Tbsp. Fresh Lemon Juice
- ¼ C. Chicken Stock
- 2 Tbsp. Coconut Aminos
- 3 Tbsp. Garlic, Finely Chopped
- 2 Tsp. Tapioca Starch
- 2 Tbsp. Water
- Red Pepper Flakes, To Taste
- Salt And Pepper

Directions

1. Put the chicken in a slow cooker.
2. Combine the honey, lemon juice, vinegar, coconut aminos, garlic, and chicken stock in a bowl and season it to taste.
3. Pour the sauce over the chicken and cook on low for six to eight hours.
4. Take the chicken out and pour the sauce into a saucepan.
5. Warm the sauce over high heat.
6. Combine two tablespoons of water with the starch and add it to the sauce. Let it come to a boil and stir as it thickens.

7. Season with the red pepper flakes and pour the sauce over the chicken. Serve on steamed vegetables.

Chicken Caesar Burgers

Serves: 4

Ingredients

- 1 Lb. Ground Chicken
- ½ Tbsp. Capers, Chopped
- 2 Tbsp. Onion, Finely Chopped
- 1 Clove Garlic, Finely Chopped
- ½ Tbsp. Fresh Parsley, Finely Chopped
- ½ Tbsp. Coconut Aminos
- Salt And Pepper To Taste
- Cooking Fat
- Tomato, Sliced Thinly
- Romaine Lettuce Leaves
- Red Onion, Sliced Thinly
- 1 C. Mayonnaise
- 3 Tbsp. Lemon Juice
- 2 Cloves Garlic, Finely Chopped
- 2 Anchovy Fillets, Chopped
- 2 Tsp. Dijon Mustard
- Pepper To Taste

Directions

1. Combine the mayonnaise through the pepper in a food processor and pulse until smooth.
2. Put in a bowl and store in the refrigerator.

3. Gently mix the ground chicken through the salt and pepper together in a bowl and make four patties.
4. Heat a grill with cooking fat over high heat.
5. Cook the patties four to five minutes on either side.
6. Serve the burgers on the lettuce, top with dressing, tomato slices, and onion.
7. Store any leftover dressing in the refrigerator up to a week.

Queso Chicken Chili in the Slow Cooker

Serves: 4

Ingredients

- 1 Lb. Boneless Skinless Chicken Breasts
- 1 Red Onion, Chopped
- 3 Bell Peppers, Finely Chopped
- 1 Jalapeño Pepper, Finely Chopped
- 2 C. Salsa
- 2 Cloves Of Garlic, Finely Chopped
- 1½ C. Water
- 2 Tsp. Chili Powder
- 1 Tsp. Ground Cumin
- 1 Avocado, Chopped
- Salt And Pepper

Directions

1. In the slow cooker, add the chicken, salsa, garlic, cumin, water, chili powder, onion, and season to taste.
2. Cover and cook on low eight hours.
3. Remove the chicken. Shred it with a fork and return it to the slow cooker.
4. Put the jalapeno and bell peppers in a skillet over high heat and cook five minutes.
5. Add the peppers to the slow cooker.
6. Let the chili simmer another twenty minutes and add water if it's necessary.

7. Top with the avocado before serving.

Chicken With Buffalo Ranch Coleslaw
Serves: 4

Ingredients
- 1 Large Carrot, Finely Shredded
- 1 Head Green Cabbage, Finely Shredded
- 4 Boneless Skinless Chicken Breasts
- 1 Tbsp. Smoked Paprika
- ½ Tbsp. Garlic Powder
- Salt And Pepper
- ¼ C. Homemade Mayonnaise
- ¼ C. Coconut Milk
- 1 Tsp. Raw Garlic, Finely Chopped
- 2 Tsp. Fresh Chives, Finely Chopped
- 2 Tsp. Fresh Dill, Finely Chopped
- ½ Tsp. Paprika
- 2 Tbsp. Hot Cayenne Pepper Sauce
- 2 Tbsp. Apple Cider Vinegar
- Salt And Pepper

Directions
1. Preheat the grill to high.
2. Combine the mayonnaise through the salt and pepper in a bowl.
3. In another bowl, combine the carrot, cabbage, and ranch sauce. Cover and keep cold.

4. In another bowl, combine the garlic powder, paprika, and salt and pepper to taste.
5. Coat the chicken with the seasoning.
6. Cook on the grill twelve minutes on either side.
7. Top the chicken with the slaw and serve.

Spicy Sriracha Chicken Wings
Serves: 2

Ingredients

- 2 Lbs. Chicken Wings
- Salt And Pepper, To Taste
- 1 Tsp. Garlic Powder
- 1 Tbsp. Fresh Cilantro Leaves, Finely Chopped
- 5 Tbsp. Olive Oil
- ¼ C. Raw Honey
- ¼ C. Sriracha Sauce
- Juice Of 1 Lime
- 1 Tbsp. Coconut Aminos

Directions

1. Preheat the oven to 400 degrees.
2. In a bowl, combine the oil, sriracha, honey, lime juice, and coconut aminos.
3. Arrange the wings on a parchment paper covered baking sheet and bake half an hour. Flip the halfway through.
4. Brush the wings with the sauce and put them under the broiler for four minutes.
5. Serve garnished with cilantro.

Butter Chicken
Serves: 4

Ingredients

- Butter
- 2.25 Lbs. Chicken, Cubed
- 2 Tsp. Garam Masala
- 2 Tsp. Ground Coriander
- 2 Tsp. Paprika
- 1 Tbsp. Grated Fresh Ginger
- ¼ Tsp Chili Powder
- 1 Cinnamon Stick
- 6 Cardamon Pods
- 1 Can Of Tomato Puree
- ¾ C. Coconut Milk
- 1 Tbsp. Fresh Lemon Juice

Directions

1. Heat the pan and add two tablespoons of butter. Stir fry the chicken.
2. Remove the chicken.
3. Put another two tablespoons of butter in the pan and heat the spices.
4. Put the chicken back in and stir.
5. Add the tomatoes and simmer fifteen minutes.
6. Add the lemon juice and coconut milk and simmer for another five minutes.
7. Enjoy.

Coconut Crusted Chicken Strips
Serves: 2-4

Ingredients

- 2 Boneless, Skinless Chicken Breasts
- ½ C. Coconut Flour
- 2 Eggs
- ¼ C. Full-Fat Coconut Milk
- 1 C. Shredded Coconut
- Salt And Pepper

Directions

1. Preheat the oven to 400 degrees.
2. Use a rolling pin to flatten the chicken breasts. Cut them into strips about an inch wide.
3. Put the coconut flour in a bowl, the coconut milk and egg in a bowl, and the shredded coconut in a bowl.
4. Coat the chicken strips in the flour, egg mix, and shredded coconut. Put them on a baking sheet and cook for twelve minutes.
5. Serve with chili sauce.

Olive, Garlic & Lemon Chicken

Serves: 4

Ingredients

- ¼ C. Butter
- ½ Lb. Kalamata Olives, Pitted, Halved
- 8 Whole Chicken Thighs
- 3 C. Onions, Sliced Thin
- 3 Gloves Garlic, Minced
- ½ C. Lemon Juice
- 2 Lemons, Thickly Sliced
- 1 ½ C. Chicken Stock
- 1 Tsp. Thyme
- Salt And Pepper

Directions

1. Preheat the oven to 350 degrees.
2. Melt the first quarter cup of fat in a hot pan and brown the chicken on all sides, about six minutes.
3. Sauté the onions three minutes.
4. Sauté the garlic a minute. Season with salt and pepper.
5. Add the stock, lemon juice, and thyme and return the thighs to the pan.
6. Bring to a simmer and put the pan in the oven, covered, for twenty minutes.
7. Remove the lid and add the olives, as well as the extra lemon slices and bake another twenty minutes, uncovered.

8. Serve the chicken with the garlic, olive, and lemon sauce and some of the lemon slices.

Baked Chicken Nuggets

Serves: 4

Ingredients

- 4 Boneless, Skinless Chicken Breasts
- 1 ½ C. Of Almond Flour
- 2 Eggs
- 1 ½ C. Of Coconut Flour
- 1 Tsp. Garlic Powder
- 1 Tsp. Dried Oregano
- 1 Tsp. Paprika
- Salt And Pepper To Taste
- 1 C. Of Homemade Mayonnaise
- 2 Cloves Of Garlic, Finely Chopped
- 1 Tbsp. Fresh Chives, Finely Chopped
- 1 Tbsp. Fresh Dill, Finely Chopped
- Salt And Pepper To Taste

Directions

1. Preheat the oven to 400 degrees.
2. Flatten the chicken with a rolling pin.
3. Combine the flours, garlic, paprika, salt and pepper, and oregano in a bowl.
4. In another bowl, whisk the eggs.
5. Dip the chicken into the eggs and coat with the flour mix. Line up on a greased baking sheet.
6. When they're coated, bake for twelve minutes.

7. As the nuggets cook, combine the mayonnaise through the salt and pepper in a bowl.
8. Serve the nuggets with the ranch and dill dip.

Pork

Pork Chops With Garlic Sage Butter
Serves: 4

Ingredients
- 4 Bone-In Pork Rib Chops
- 4 Cloves Of Garlic, Smashed
- 8 Sprigs Sage
- 4 Tbsp. Ghee
- Cooking Fat
- Salt And Pepper

Directions
1. Melt the fat in a skillet over high heat.
2. Season the chops to taste on either side.
3. Put the chops in the skillet and cook ten minutes. Turning every minute.
4. Remove from the skillet and add the ghee, garlic, and sage.
5. Let the butter melt and mix it with the garlic and sage.
6. Let the skillet sit for four minutes. Baste the pork chops with the butter mix.

Pork Tenderloin With Warm Pear Salsa
Serves: 4

Ingredients

- 1 Pork Tenderloin
- 1 Onion, Chopped
- 2 Pears, Chopped
- 2 Cloves Of Garlic
- ¼ C. Walnuts, Chopped
- 3 Tbsp. Balsamic Vinegar
- 1 Tbsp. Fresh Chives, Finely Chopped
- 1 Tbsp. Fresh Lemon Juice
- ½ C. Chicken Stock
- Cooking Fat
- Salt And Pepper

Directions

1. Preheat the oven to 400 degrees.
2. Combine the walnut, pear, chives, lemon juice, and salt and pepper in a bowl.
3. Melt some fat in a skillet over high heat.
4. Brown the tenderloin on all sides, three minutes on every side.
5. Lower the heat to medium and add the onion and garlic. Cook until fragrant, around two minutes.
6. Pour in the vinegar and bring it to a boil as you stir and scrape the browned bits up from the pan.

7. Add the chicken stock.
8. Drizzle the pear salsa over the tenderloin and bake for twenty minutes.
9. Let it rest five minutes before slicing and serving with the salsa.

Maple-Barbecue Ribs
Serves: 4

Ingredients
- 4 Lb. Pork Back Ribs
- 1 Tbsp. Onion Powder
- 1 Tbsp. Smoked Paprika
- ½ Tsp. Ground Chili Flakes
- ½ Tbsp. Onion Powder
- 2 Tsp. Ground Cumin
- Salt And Pepper
- 1 C. Homemade Ketchup
- 1 C. Apple Juice
- ▯ C. Maple Syrup
- ¼ C. Apple Cider Vinegar
- 2 Cloves Of Garlic, Finely Chopped
- 1 Onion, Finely Chopped
- Cooking Fat
- Salt And Pepper

Directions
1. Combine the paprika, ground cumin, onion powder, and chili flakes in a bowl. Season to taste.
2. Rub the ribs with the spice mix and put in a marinating container for two to twelve hours in the fridge.
3. Preheat the oven to 300 degrees.

4. Wrap the ribs with foil and put them on a baking sheet. Bake for two hours.
5. In a saucepan, melt the fat over medium heat and sauté the garlic and onion.
6. Add the ketchup through the apple cider vinegar and season to taste. Cook for twenty minutes.
7. Baste the ribs with the sauce and increase the temperature to 400 degrees. Return to the oven and bake another twenty minutes, basting every five minutes with the sauce.
8. Brown the ribs on either side for five minutes under the broiler before serving.

Pork Chops with Vinaigrette

Serves: 4

Ingredients

- 4 Bone-In Pork Chops
- ½ C. Extra-Virgin Olive Oil
- ¼ C. Fresh Lemon Juice
- ¼ C. Fresh Orange Juice
- 2 Cloves Garlic, Finely Chopped
- 2 Tbsp. Fresh Cilantro Finely Chopped
- ½ Tsp. Red Pepper Flakes
- Salt And Pepper

Directions

1. Preheat the grill to medium high.
2. Whisk the lemon and orange juice together with the garlic, oil, red pepper flakes, and the cilantro.
3. Season the chops to taste with the salt and pepper.
4. Put the chops on the grill and cook for five minutes on either side. Let them rest three minutes.
5. Serve drizzled with the vinaigrette.

Pork Chops With Balsamic Glaze
Serves: 4

Ingredients
- 4 Boneless Pork Chops
- ¼ C. Balsamic Vinegar
- 3 Tbsp. Raw Honey
- 2 Cloves Of Garlic, Finely Chopped
- ½ Tsp. Dried Oregano
- ½ Tsp. Dried Thyme
- ½ Tsp. Dried Basil
- 1 Tsp. Crushed Red Pepper Flakes
- Salt And Pepper

Directions
1. Preheat the oven to 400 degrees.
2. Season the chops to taste with salt and pepper.
3. In a pan, combine the vinegar, garlic, honey, basil, oregano, red pepper flakes, thyme, and salt and pepper.
4. Bring it to a boil and reduce the heat to a simmer for five minutes.
5. Sear the chops on either side in a skillet over high heat, two minutes per side.
6. Brush the chops with the glaze and transfer the skillet to the oven and roast eight minutes.
7. Brush them a last time with the glaze before serving.

Cinnamon Pork Chops with Spiced Pear Chutney

Serves: 4

Ingredients

- 4 To 6 Pork Chops, Bone-In
- 2 Tsp. Ground Cinnamon
- 2 Tbsp. Chili Powder
- 2 Tsp. Garlic Powder
- Salt And Pepper
- 2 Tsp. Onion Powder
- 3 Pears, Peeled, And Chopped
- ▯ C. Apple Cider Vinegar
- ¼ C. Raw Honey
- ½ Tsp. Ground Ginger
- ½ Tsp. Ground Cinnamon
- ½ Tsp. Chili Powder
- ¼ Tsp. Ground Nutmeg
- Salt And Pepper

Directions

1. Preheat the grill to medium heat.
2. Mix the chili powder, garlic powder, cinnamon, and onion together for the chops and season with salt and pepper.
3. Rub the chops with the spice mix until they're coated.
4. Combine the pear through the salt and pepper in a saucepan.

5. Cook the chutney for ten minutes over medium heat.
6. Grill the chops five minutes on either side and allow them to rest four minutes.
7. Serve with the pear chutney.

Ham And Butternut Squash Hash
Serves: 4

Ingredients
- 1 Butternut Squash, Peeled And Cubed
- 2 C. Pre-Cooked Ham, Cubed
- 1 Leek, Sliced
- 1 Onion, Sliced
- 1 Green Apple, Peeled And Cubed
- 2 Cloves Of Garlic, Finely Chopped
- 1 Tsp. Ground Cinnamon
- 1 Tsp. Paprika
- Cooking Fat
- Salt And Pepper

Directions
1. Melt the fat in a skillet over high heat.
2. Sauté the onion and garlic three minutes.
3. Add the squash and leek and cook seven minutes.
4. Add the apple and ham and warm it through.
5. Season with the paprika, cinnamon, and salt and pepper.
6. Cook another two minutes before serving.

Ham and Pineapple Skewers
Serves: 4

Ingredients
- 1 Pineapple, Cut Into Cubes
- 1 Lb. Ham, Cut Into Cubes
- ¼ C. Fresh Pineapple Juice
- 1 Tsp. Dijon Mustard
- 2 Tsp. Raw Honey
- 2 Tsp. Coconut Aminos
- ½ Tbsp. Fresh Ginger, Finely Chopped
- Salt And Pepper
- Wood Or Metal Skewers

Directions
1. Preheat the grill to high heat.
2. In a bowl, add the coconut aminos, pineapple juice, ginger, honey, and mustard and season to taste.
3. Thread pieces of ham and pineapple onto the skewers.
4. Grill the skewers for ten minutes, basting and turning frequently.

Pork Tenderloin With Strawberry Sauce
Serves: 4

Ingredients
- 4 Lbs. Pork Tenderloin
- 10 Bacon Slices
- 1 C. Strawberries, Sliced
- ½ C. Balsamic Vinegar
- 4 Cloves Of Garlic, Finely Chopped
- Olive Oil
- Salt And Pepper

Directions
1. Preheat the grill to high.
2. Wrap the bacon around the tenderloin and secure it.
3. Put the tenderloin on the grill and cook for half an hour, turning occasionally.
4. Heat the oil in a saucepan over high heat and sauté the garlic two minutes.
5. Add the vinegar and half a cup of the strawberries and bring it to a boil.
6. Lower the heat to a simmer for ten minutes.
7. Season the sauce to taste and add the rest of the strawberries.
8. Baste the tenderloin with the sauce and cook over direct heat until the bacon is crispy.

9. Slice the pork and serve with the rest of the sauce.

Pulled Pork With Mustard Sauce and Barbecue Sauce
Serves: 4

Ingredients
- 4 Lbs. Pork Shoulder
- 1 C. Old Fashioned Mustard
- ¼ C. Raw Honey
- ¼ C. Apple Cider Vinegar
- 2 Tsp. Hot Pepper Sauce
- 1 Tbsp. Coconut Aminos
- Salt And Pepper
- 2 Tbsp. Paprika
- ½ Tbsp. Onion Powder
- ½ Tbsp. Garlic Powder
- ½ Tbsp. Chili Powder
- Salt And Pepper
- ½ Tbsp. Ground Cumin

Directions
1. Combine the paprika through the ground cumin in a bowl.
2. Rub the spice mix over the pork shoulder and put it in a slow cooker.
3. In another bowl, mix the mustard, vinegar, honey, hot pepper sauce, and coconut aminos together. Season to taste.
4. Pour the sauce over the pork and cook on low for eight hours.

5. Shred the pork and remove any large hunks of fat.
6. Stir the pork in the sauce to mix it and serve.

Seafood

Grilled Scallop And Orange Skewers
Serves: 4

Ingredients
- 1 Navel Orange, Sliced, And Segmented
- 12 Sea Scallops
- 1 Tbsp. Fresh Ginger, Finely Chopped
- Juice From 1 Orange
- 2 Tbsp. Olive Oil
- 2 Tbsp. Fresh Lemon Juice
- Salt And Pepper
- Wood Or Metal Skewers

Directions
1. Preheat the grill to medium heat.
2. Combine the lemon and orange juice in a bowl with the olive oil and ginger.
3. Thread the orange slices and scallops onto the skewers.
4. Season to taste.
5. Brush with the orange juice sauce.
6. Grill for two to three minutes on either side, basting constantly.
7. Serve on lettuce.

Spicy Mussel Soup
Serves: 4

Ingredients

- 2 Lbs. Mussels, Prepared
- 2 Shallots, Finely Chopped
- 2 Cloves Of Garlic, Finely Chopped
- 3 C. Fish Or Vegetable Stock
- 2 C. Coconut Milk
- 3 Tbsp. Chili Paste
- 1 Tbsp. Fresh Lemon Juice
- 1 Tsp. Dried Chili Flakes
- 3 Fresh Thai Basil Leaves
- ½ Dry White Wine
- Cooking Fat
- Fresh Cilantro, Finely Chopped
- Salt And Pepper

Directions

1. Melt the fat in a skillet over medium heat.
2. Cook the garlic and shallots until they're soft.
3. Pour the white wine in. Bring it to a boil and allow it to simmer until it reduces to half.
4. Add the fish stock, chili paste, coconut milk, basil, chili, lemon juice and salt and pepper. Lower the heat and simmer ten minutes.

5. Add the mussels and cook five minutes or until they open fully.
6. Serve with the sauce and garnish with cilantro.

Spicy Tuna And Cucumber Bites
Serves: 4

Ingredients

- ½ Lb. Tuna (Sushi Grade), Finely Chopped
- 1 Cucumber, Sliced Into Thin Rounds
- 1 Avocado, Thinly Cubed
- 1 Green Onion, Finely Sliced
- 2 Tbsp. Coconut Aminos
- 1 Tsp. Sesame Seeds
- 2 Tsp. Sriracha Sauce
- Salt And Pepper

Directions

1. In a bowl, add the coconut aminos, tuna, sriracha sauce, and salt and pepper. Toss.
2. Top the cucumber slices with an avocado slice.
3. Scoop the tuna mix onto the cucumber slices.
4. Sprinkle with the sesames seeds and garnish with green onions.

Smoked Salmon With Fresh Vegetables
Serves: 2

Ingredients

- 8 Oz. Smoked Salmon, Cut Into Thin Slices
- 2 C. Grape Tomatoes, Halved
- 1 Red Onion, Thinly Sliced
- 1 Cucumber, Peeled And Coarsely Chopped
- 6 Tbsp. Olive Oil
- ½ Tsp. Garlic, Finely Chopped
- 2 Tbsp. Fresh Lemon Juice
- 1 Tsp. Balsamic Vinegar
- ½ Tsp. Dried Oregano
- Fresh Dill, Finely Chopped
- Salt And Pepper

Directions

1. In a bowl, whisk the olive oil, garlic, lemon juice, vinegar, and oregano together.
2. Season the dressing to taste.
3. Combine the cucumber, tomatoes, and onion in a bowl.
4. Drizzle with the dressing and toss.
5. Roll the smoke salmon slices up and put them on the fresh vegetables.
6. Sprinkle with the dill and serve.

Pistachio-Crusted Salmon
Serves: 4

Ingredients
- 4 Wild Salmon Fillets
- 1 C. Raw Pistachios, Roughly Chopped
- ¼ C. Lemon Juice
- 2 Tbsp. Raw Honey
- 1 Tbsp. Dijon
- 1 Tsp. Fresh Dill Weed
- Salt And Pepper

Directions
1. Preheat your oven to 375 degrees.
2. Combine the lemon juice, pistachio, mustard, dill, and honey in a bowl and season to taste.
3. Spread the pistachio mix over the salmon filets and press it to make it stick.
4. Bake the salmon, uncovered, twenty minutes.
5. Let it rest four minutes before serving.

Fried Fish Tacos
Serves: 4

Ingredients

- 1 ½ Lbs. Tilapia Fillets
- 1 ¼ C. Tapioca Starch
- ¼ C. Coconut Flour
- 2 Eggs
- ¼ C. Sparkling Water
- 2 C. Coconut Oil For Frying
- 2 C. Cabbage, Shredded
- Lime Wedges, For Serving
- Cauliflower Tortillas
- Salt And Pepper
- 2 Roma Tomatoes, Chopped
- ¼ C. Onion, Finely Chopped
- 1 Tbsp. Fresh Cilantro, Chopped
- 2 Tbsp. Jalapeño, Finely Chopped
- 2 Tbsp. Freshly Squeezed Lime Juice
- Sea Salt
- ¼ C. Homemade Mayonnaise
- 1 Tbsp. Homemade Sriracha
- 2 Tsp. Lime Juice

Directions

1. Mix the onion, tomatoes, cilantro, and jalapenos together.
2. Add the lime juice and a little salt.
3. Taste and adjust if necessary.

4. Cover and refrigerate.
5. Mix the final three ingredients together to make the spicy mayonnaise.
6. Cover and refrigerate until ready to serve.
7. Heat the coconut oil in a saucepan until it reaches 345 degrees. Be sure to keep the oil ten degrees below the smoking point.
8. Mix three quarters of a cup of the starch with the eggs, coconut flour, sparkling water, and salt and pepper to taste in a bowl.
9. Put half a cup of the starch in another bowl.
10. Trim the fish into pieces.
11. Once the oil's ready, pat the tilapia dry and coat with the starch. Shake off any excess.
12. Put the coated fish into the batter mix and use tongs to lift it up and let any excess batter drip off.
13. Immediately put it in the oil and let it fry a minute. Turn it over and cook another minute.
14. Once it's cooked, remove it from the oil and put it on a paper towel to absorb the cooking oil.
15. Cut the fillets in half to assemble the tacos. Put a small amount of cabbage eon the tortilla, then layer the fish, Pico de Gallo, and spicy mayo in the taco.

Buffalo Shrimp Recipe

Serves: 4

Ingredients

- 1 Lb. Shrimp, Peeled And Deveined
- 1 Clove Of Garlic, Finely Chopped
- 4 C. Mixed Greens
- ▯ C. Buffalo Sauce
- 1 Cucumber, Sliced
- 1 Small Red Onion, Sliced
- 6 Oz. Cherry Tomatoes, Halved
- Cooking Fat

Directions

1. Melt the fat in the skillet over medium heat.
2. Add the garlic and shrimp and sauté for five minutes.
3. Add the buffalo sauce, and cook another two minutes.
4. Serve the shrimp over the salad greens topped with tomatoes, cucumber, and onion.
5. Drizzle the sauce over the top.

Fennel and Lemon Roasted Trout

Serves: 4

Ingredients

- 3 Rainbow Trout, Prepared
- 2 Lemons, Thinly Sliced
- 1 Bunch Fresh Rosemary
- 1 Bunch Fresh Dill
- 2 Tbsp. Olive Oil
- 2 Fennel Bulbs, Cut Into Slices
- Salt And Pepper

Directions

1. Preheat the oven to 500 degrees.
2. Grease a baking pan.
3. Arrange the fennel on a single layer on the baking pan.
4. Season the trout with salt and pepper.
5. Put the fish on top of the fennel on the baking pan.
6. Fill the fish cavity with lemon slices, rosemary, and dill.
7. Top the fish with the leftover lemon slices and herbs.
8. Put the baking pan in the oven and cook ten minutes.
9. Lower the heat to 425 degrees and cook ten to twelve minutes.

Asian Marinated Tuna with Shaved Salad
Serves: 4

Ingredients
- 4 Tuna Steaks, About 6 Oz. Each
- ¼ C. Olive Oil
- 2 Tbsp. Coconut Aminos
- 2 Tbsp. Lime Juice
- 2 Tbsp. Rice Vinegar
- 1 Tbsp. Fresh Ginger, Grated
- 3 Tbsp. Cooking Fat
- 2 Cloves Of Garlic, Finely Chopped
- Salt And Pepper
- 6 Carrots, Peeled
- 1 English Cucumber, Peeled
- 1 Bunch Asparagus, Ends Trimmed
- ½ C. Coconut Aminos
- 1 Tbsp. Rice Vinegar
- 3 Tbsp. Lemon Juice
- 2 Tsp. Green Onion, Finely Chopped
- 1 Tsp. Fresh Ginger, Grated

Directions
1. Make the marinade by combining the olive oil, rice vinegar, coconut aminos, ginger, lime juice, and garlic in a plastic bag.
2. Season the tuna with salt and pepper on the sides then put them in the marinade.

Turn to coat and refrigerate for half an hour. Turn halfway through.

3. Whisk the lemon juice, coconut aminos, green onion, vinegar, and ginger to make the dressing for the salad. Set it aside.

4. Use a peeler to shave the asparagus, carrots, and cucumber in long strips. For the carrot and cucumber, rotate them as you peel.

5. Put the ribbons in a bowl and coat with the dressing, around half, and toss to mix. Reserve the rest of the dressing.

6. Heat the skillet over medium heat.

7. Sear the tuna steak for two minutes on either side. Divide the shaved salad on four plates and top with the tuna steak. Serve with the reserved dressing.

Maple Salmon With Chives and Dill

Serves: 4

Ingredients

- 4 Salmon Filets, 6 Oz. Each
- 2 Tbsp. Dill, Finely Chopped
- 2 Tbsp. Chives, Finely Chopped
- ▯ C. Maple Syrup
- 3 Tbsp. White Balsamic Vinegar
- Cooking Fat
- Salt And Pepper
- Lime Wedges

Directions

1. Melt the fat in a skillet over medium heat.
2. Season the fish to taste.
3. Cook the fillets in the skillet with the skin side down for two to three minutes. Cover and cook another six minutes.
4. Add the maple syrup and the vinegar to the skillet and cook for three minutes. Baste the fish with the sauce for the rest of the cooking time.
5. Sprinkle the chopped chives and dill over the filets and serve with the lime wedges.

Soups

Basic Vegetable Soup
Serves: 4

Ingredients

- 2 C. Kale, Chopped And With The Stems Removed
- 2 C. Red Cabbage, Chopped
- 1 Red Onion, Chopped
- 4 Carrots, Chopped
- 3 Celery Stalks, Chopped
- 1 Head Of Broccoli, Cut Into Florets
- 1 Tbsp. Fresh Ginger, Finely Chopped
- 1 C. Grape Tomatoes, Halved
- 2 Cloves Of Garlic, Finely Chopped
- ¼ Tsp. Ground Cinnamon
- 1 Tsp. Ground Turmeric
- 6 C. Vegetable Stock
- Salt And Pepper

Directions

1. Add the ginger, onion, and garlic to a pan over medium heat.
2. Sauté for two to three minutes.
3. Add the carrots, celery, and tomatoes. Stir to mix and cook three to five minutes.
4. Stir in the cinnamon, turmeric, and salt and pepper it to taste.

5. Add the cabbage, broccoli, and vegetable broth and bring it to a boil.
6. Reduce the heat and simmer fifteen minutes.
7. Add the kale three minutes before serving to wilt.

Winter Pumpkin Soup with Curry Spices

Serves: 4

Ingredients

- 1 Pumpkin, Halved And Seeded
- 2 Russet, Chopped
- 1 Onion, Chopped
- 1 Carrot, Chopped
- 2 Garlic Clove, Finely Chopped
- 1 Tsp. Ginger, Finely Chopped
- ¼ Tsp. Coriander Powder
- ½ Tsp. Curry Powder
- 4 C. Vegetable Stock
- 2 Tbsp. Fresh Lime Juice
- Cooking Fat
- Salt And Pepper

Directions

1. Preheat the oven to 400 degrees.
2. Put the pumpkin halves upside down on a baking sheet with some parchment paper.
3. Bake about forty minutes.
4. With a spoon, scrape the flesh from the skin and put it in a bowl. Puree with an immersion blender.
5. Melt some fat in a pan over medium heat.
6. Add the onion and garlic and cook for three minutes.

7. Add the carrot and potato chunks and pour in the stock. Bring to a boil.
8. Lower the heat until the vegetables are tender.
9. Mash with a potato masher.
10. Add the pumpkin and the rest of the ingredients. Season to taste. Give it a good stir.
11. Puree with an immersion blender.
12. Let the soup simmer and warm.

Directions

1. Put the turkey carcass and the parts in a saucepan and add the celery through the pepper. Season to taste.
2. Fill the pan with water and bring it to a boil.
3. Lower the heat and simmer for eight hours.
4. Strain the stock and throw away the rest of the ingredients. Set aside the stock.
5. Pick through the carcass and remove the meat you find. Add the meat to a pot.
6. Add all the ingredients for the soup into a pan and fill the pan with turkey stock. Season to taste.
7. Simmer for forty-five minutes to an hour.

Cauliflower Chowder

Serves: 4

Ingredients

- 1 Head Cauliflower, Roughly Chopped
- 2 Celery Stalks, Chopped
- 1 Onion, Chopped
- 2 Cloves Of Garlic, Finely Chopped
- 2 Carrots, Peeled And Chopped
- 4 C. Chicken Stock
- 1 C. Coconut Milk
- 1 Tsp. Ground Turmeric
- 1¼ Tsp. Ground Cumin
- ½ Tsp. Ground Coriander
- Fresh Dill, To Taste
- 4 Bacon Slices, Cooked And Crumbled
- Cooking Fat
- Salt And Pepper

Directions

1. Melt the fat in a large saucepan and put it over medium heat.
2. Add the onion, garlic, celery, and carrots, and cook five minutes.
3. Stir in the cauliflower and cook for five minutes.
4. Add in the chicken stock, turmeric, cumin, coconut milk, coriander, and stir together.

5. Bring to a boil and reduce for fifteen minutes.
6. Season to taste and serve garnished with bacon and dill.

Slow Cooker Sweet Potato Soup

Serves: 4

Ingredients

- 3 Lbs. Sweet Potatoes, Chopped
- 2 Stalks Celery, Sliced
- 1 Onion, Chopped
- 2 Carrots, Chopped
- 5 C. Chicken Or Vegetable Stock
- 1 Tbsp. Garlic, Finely Chopped
- 1 C. Coconut Milk
- Salt And Pepper

Directions

1. Put everything in the slow cooker but the coconut milk.
2. Season to taste.
3. Cover and cook on low six hours.
4. Puree until smooth with an immersion blender.
5. Add the milk, give it a good stir, and cook for half an hour.
6. Adjust the seasoning and serve warm.

Wild Mushroom Soup

Serves: 4

Ingredients

- 2 Large Shallots, Chopped
- 1 ½ Lb. Mixed Wild Mushrooms, Sliced
- 1 Tbsp. Fresh Thyme
- 7 C. Chicken Stock
- 3 Tbsp. Ghee
- 1 C. Coconut Milk
- ¼ C. Parsley, Chopped
- 2 Tbsp. Tapioca Starch
- Salt And Pepper

Directions

1. Melt the ghee in a saucepan over medium high heat.
2. Sauté the shallots for four minutes.
3. Add the thyme and mushrooms and cook eight minutes.
4. Add the stock and bring it to a boil. Turn down the heat and simmer fifteen minutes.
5. Stir in the coconut milk, season, and allow it to simmer five minutes.
6. Stir in the starch.
7. Mix in the parsley and serve.

Slow Cooker Beef And Pepper Soup

Serves: 4

Ingredients

- 1 Lb. Extra-Lean Ground Beef
- 1 C. Onion, Chopped
- 2 C. Cauliflower, Finely Chopped
- 2 Bell Peppers, Chopped
- 15 Oz. Tomato Sauce
- 15 Oz. Chopped Tomatoes
- 3 C. Beef Stock
- ½ Tsp. Dried Oregano
- ½ Tsp. Dried Basil
- 3 Cloves Garlic, Crushed
- Cooking Fat
- Salt And Pepper

Directions

1. Melt the fat in a skillet over high heat and sauté the onions and garlic a minute.
2. Add the beef and cook until the meat has browned.
3. Put the beef and onion mix in a slow cooker.
4. Add the rest of the ingredients, season, and give it a good stir.
5. Cover and cook six to eight hours.

Old Fashioned Cabbage Soup
Serves: 4

Ingredients
- 2 Chicken Breasts, Cut Into Chunks
- 1 Leek, Sliced
- 2 Celery Stalks, Sliced
- 2 Carrots, Sliced
- 2 Sweet Potatoes, Chopped
- 1 C. Rutabaga, Chopped
- 3 C. Shredded Cabbage
- 8 C. Chicken Stock
- 2 Cloves Of Garlic, Finely Chopped
- Cooking Fat
- Salt And Pepper

Directions
1. Melt the fat in a saucepan over medium heat.
2. Add the chicken and garlic and cook five minutes.
3. Add the celery, carrots and leek and cook another four minutes
4. Add the rest of the ingredients, season to taste, and stir.
5. Cover and cook twenty minutes, or until soft.

Coconut Lime Chicken Soup
Serves: 4

Ingredients
- 2 Lbs. Cooked Chicken, Cut Into Pieces
- 15 Oz. Coconut Milk
- 3 C. Chicken Broth
- ¼ C. Lime Juice
- 1 C. Broccoli, Shredded
- 3 Medium Carrots, Shredded
- 1 C. Rutabaga, Shredded
- 1 Lime Cut Into Wedges
- Salt And Pepper
- ½ Tsp. Curry Powder
- ¼ Tsp. Ginger
- ¼ Tsp. Cinnamon
- ¼ Tsp. Chili Powder
- ¼ Tsp. Salt
- ¼ Tsp. Paprika

Directions
1. Combine the broth, milk, lime juice, curry powder through paprika, shredded vegetables, and chicken pieces in a saucepan. Season to taste.
2. Bring to a boil, reduce the heat and simmer fifteen minutes.
3. Serve warm with the lime wedges.

Chunky Meat and Vegetable Soup

Serves: 4

Ingredients

- 2-½ Lbs. Ground Beef
- 1 Large Onion, Chopped
- 3 Cloves Of Garlic, Finely Chopped
- 2 Celery Stalks, Chopped
- 14.5 Oz. Can Of Chopped Tomatoes
- 3 C. Beef Broth
- 3 Bell Peppers, Seeded And Chopped
- 2 Sweet Potatoes, Cut Into Chunks
- 4 Whole Carrots, Peeled And Sliced
- 3 Tbsp. Tomato Paste
- 1 Tsp. Chili Powder
- ½ Tsp. Ground Oregano
- Salt And Pepper

Directions

1. Brown the meat, onion, celery, and garlic in a saucepan over medium heat.
2. Add the rest of the ingredients and season to taste. Stir to combine.
3. Bring to a boil, reduce to a simmer, and cook twenty minutes or until the potatoes are soft.

Salads

Avocado, Apple And Chicken Salad
Serves: 4

Ingredients
- 2 C. Cooked Chicken, Finely Chopped
- 1 Apple, Peeled, Cored, And Finely Chopped
- 1 Avocado, Seeded, Peeled, And Chopped
- ¼ C. Celery, Finely Chopped
- ¼ C. Red Onion, Finely Chopped
- 2 Tbsp. Extra-Virgin Olive Oil
- 2 Tbsp. Fresh Parsley, Finely Chopped
- 2 Tsp. Fresh Lime Juice
- ½ Tsp. Garlic Powder
- Salt And Pepper

Directions
1. In a bowl, whisk the oil, garlic, lime juice, and parsley together. Season to taste.
2. Combine the rest of the ingredients in the bowl.
3. Pour the dressing over the chicken and avocado mix.
4. Toss until its coated.

5. Serve as a salad or wrapped in lettuce.

Cranberry And Clementine Salad
Serves: 4

Ingredients
- 2.5 Oz. Baby Kale
- 2.5 Oz. Fresh Spinach
- ¾ C. Celery, Chopped
- ¾ C. Dried Cranberries
- 4 Eggs
- 2 Clementines, Segmented
- 1 Apple, Cored And Sliced
- ¼ C. Pine Nuts, Roasted
- ¼ C. Extra-Virgin Olive Oil
- 2 Tbsp. Apple Cider Vinegar
- ⅛ Tsp. Paprika
- 1 Tbsp. Fresh Lemon Juice
- ⅛ Tsp. Onion Powder
- 1 Tbsp. Poppy Seeds

Directions
1. Bring a pan filled with water to a boil.
2. Carefully add the eggs and cover. Remove them from the heat and let them cook ten minutes.
3. Put the eggs in a bowl of ice water for three minutes.
4. Peel and slice the eggs.

5. Combine the olive oil through the poppy seeds in a b owl and whisk until emulsified.
6. In another bowl, combine the kale, spinach, celery, apple, cranberries, and oranges.
7. Drizzle with the dressing and toss until coated.
8. Put the sliced eggs on the top and garnish with pine nuts before serving.

Chicken And Avocado Caesar Salad

Serves: 4

Ingredients

- 1 Head Romaine Lettuce
- 1 Avocado, Sliced
- 2 Chicken Breasts, Skinless And Boneless
- 4 Bacon Slices, Diced And Crumbled
- 2 Eggs, Boiled And Sliced
- ½ Tbsp. Garlic Powder
- ½ Tbsp. Chili Powder
- ½ Tbsp. Dried Oregano
- Salt And Pepper
- 1 C. Homemade Mayonnaise
- 2 Cloves Of Garlic, Finely Chopped
- 2 Tsp. Anchovy Paste
- 2 Tbsp. Fresh Lemon Juice
- 1 Tsp. Dijon Mustard
- Salt And Pepper

Directions

1. Preheat the grill to high heat.
2. Rub the chicken with garlic powder, chili powder, oregano, and salt and pepper.
3. Grill the chicken six minutes on either side or until it's no longer pink.
4. Transfer to a cutting board and slice.

5. In a bowl, whisk the homemade mayonnaise through the salt and pepper together.
6. Toss the bacon, lettuce, and avocado together. Divide the mix amongst bowls and top with sliced chicken and the eggs.
7. Drizzle with the dressing and serve.

Thai-Style Steak Salad
Serves: 4

Ingredients
- 1-Lb. Skirt Steak
- 4 C. Lettuce, Chopped
- ½ English Cucumber, Sliced
- 1 Red Bell Pepper, Sliced In Long Strips
- ¼ C. Cilantro, Chopped
- ¼ C. Coconut Aminos
- ¼ C. Mint, Chopped
- 1 Tbsp. Ginger, Finely Chopped
- 3 Cloves Of Garlic, Finely Chopped
- Juice From 1 Lime
- 1 Thai Red Chili Pepper, Chopped
- Slivered Almonds
- Salt And Pepper
- 3 Tbsp. Coconut Aminos
- 2 Tbsp. Coconut Oil, Melted
- 1 Tsp. Fish Sauce
- 1 Thai Red Chili Pepper, Finely Chopped
- Zest And Juice From 1 Lime

Directions
1. Prepare the marinade by mixing the garlic, ginger, chili, coconut aminos, and lime juice together in a bowl.
2. Put the steak in a plastic bag and cover with the marinade for half an hour.

3. Combine the coconut aminos and the zest and juice of the lime. Whisk until emulsified.
4. Preheat the grill to high.
5. Grill the steak four minutes on either side on the grill.
6. Set it aside and let it rest for four minutes, then slice.
7. Toss the bell pepper, lettuce, and cucumber together.
8. Drizzle the dressing and toss.
9. Arrange the vegetables on plates and top with the sliced steak.
10. Top with the mint, cilantro, and slivered almonds.

Lobster salad With Taro Chips
Serves: 4

Ingredients

- 4 8 oz. Lobster Tails
- ▯C. Homemade Mayonnaise
- 1 Avocado, Peeled And Chopped
- ▯ C. Celery, Finely Chopped
- 3 Tbsp. Lemon Juice
- 1 ½ Tbsp. Chives, Finely Chopped
- Salt And Pepper
- Romaine Lettuce Leaves
- 1-2 Tbsp. Olive Oil
- 3 Lbs. Taro Roots, Peeled
- Salt And Pepper

Directions

1. Preheat the oven to 350 degrees.
2. Use a sharp knife to slice the taro into thin rounds.
3. Add the taro and oil in a bowl and toss to coat. Add more oil.
4. Lay the slices on a baking sheet lined with parchment paper. Season to taste.
5. Bake twenty-eight minutes in the oven and turn halfway through until they're crisp.
6. Fill a pot with salt water and bring to a boil.

7. Prepare an ice water bath to fit the lobster tails.
8. Add the lobster to the water and cook eight to ten minutes until the shells are bright red.
9. Remove the tails and immediately transfer to the ice water bath. Let it sit for two minutes. Drain.
10. Cut the tails in half to remove the meat from the shell. Cut the lobster meat into bite sized pieces. Pat dry and refrigerate ten minutes to cool.
11. Combine the celery, mayonnaise, chives, and lemon juice together. Season to taste.
12. Add the lobster to the mix and combine. Put it in the refrigerator for fifteen minutes.
13. Serve the lobster chilled over the lettuce topped with the avocado.

Shrimp And Avocado Salad
Serves: 4

Ingredients

- 2 Lbs. Steamed Shrimp, Peeled And Deveined
- 2 Avocados, Cut Into Cubes
- 2 Tbsp. Red Onion, Chopped
- Fresh Parsley, Finely Chopped
- ¼ C. Extra Virgin Olive Oil
- ¼ C. Balsamic Vinegar
- 1 Tsp. Parsley, Chopped
- ½ Tsp. Garlic Powder
- 1 Tsp. Dijon Mustard
- Salt And Pepper

Directions

1. Combine the oil through the salt and pepper together in a bowl and whisk to emulsify.
2. Toss the shrimp, avocado, and onions together.
3. Drizzle the dressing over the salad and toss.
4. Serve garnished with the parsley.

Cucumber And Strawberry Salad

Serves: 4

Ingredients

- 2 Cucumbers, Thinly Sliced
- 4 C. Strawberries, Sliced
- ¼ C. Raspberry Vinegar
- 1 Tsp. Onion, Finely Chopped
- 1 Tsp. Ground Dry Mustard
- 1 C. Extra Virgin Olive Oil
- ¼ C. Raw Honey
- 1 Tbsp. Poppy Seeds

Directions

1. Combine the oil through the poppy seeds in a bowl.
2. Toss the strawberries and cucumbers together.
3. Pour the dressing over the salad and toss.

Tomato And Spinach Salad
Serves: 4

Ingredients

- 4 Tomatoes, Quartered
- 8 Oz. Baby Spinach Leaves
- 8 Oz. Grape Tomatoes, Halved
- ¼ C. Pine Nuts, Toasted
- ¼ C. Fresh Basil, Coarsely Chopped
- ¼ C. Extra-Virgin Olive Oil
- 2 Tbsp. Balsamic Vinegar
- Salt And Pepper

Directions

1. Combine the oil and vinegar in a bowl. Stir until combined and season to taste.
2. Combine the basil, tomatoes, spinach, and nuts in a bowl.
3. Drizzle with the dressing and toss to combine.

BBQ Chicken Salad
Serves: 4

Ingredients

- 2 Boneless Skinless Chicken Breasts, Sliced Into Strips
- 6 C. Romaine Lettuce, Chopped
- 1 Bell Pepper, Cut Into Small Pieces
- 1 Roma Tomato, Chopped
- ½ Avocado, Cut Into Cubes
- ¼ C. Red Onion, Chopped
- ¼ C. Bbq Sauce
- Cooking Fat
- Salt And Pepper
- 2 Tbsp. Coconut Milk
- 2 Tbsp. Homemade Mayonnaise
- ¼ Tsp. Raw Garlic, Finely Chopped
- 1 Tsp. Fresh Chives, Finely Chopped
- 1 Tsp. Fresh Dill, Finely Chopped
- ¼ Tsp. Paprika
- Salt And Pepper

Directions

1. Add the fat to a skillet over medium high heat.
2. Season the chicken.
3. Add the chicken to the skillet and sauté for three to four minutes per side.

4. Wait until the chicken has cooled and dice it into bite-sized pieces.
5. Combine the coconut milk through the salt and pepper and whisk.
6. Fill the salad bowl with the lettuce and top with the chicken, onion, pepper, tomato, and avocado.
7. Pour the dressing and barbecue sauce on the salad. Toss to combine and serve.

Warm Winter Salad
Serves: 4

Ingredients
- 1 Butternut Squash, Cut Into Wedges
- 4 Parsnips, Cut Into Wedges
- 2 Red Onions, Cut Into Wedges
- 6 C. Of Baby Spinach
- ▯ C. Roasted Nuts
- 2 Tbsp. White Wine Vinegar
- 1 Garlic Clove, Finely Chopped
- 1 Tsp. Dijon Mustard
- ½ Tbsp. Dried Oregano
- 6 Tbsp. Extra-Virgin Olive Oil
- Salt And Pepper To Taste

Directions
1. Preheat the oven to 400 degrees.
2. Put the squash, parsnips, and onions in a baking tray. Put half the oil and the dried oregano over it and season.
3. Roast in the oven twenty minutes, turning after ten minutes.
4. Combine the oil, mustard, vinegar, and garlic together in a bowl. Season to taste.
5. Put the spinach in a bowl and add the vegetables, as well as the dressing, toss to combine.
6. Serve.

Vegetables and Sides

Sweet Potato Bites with Guacamole and Bacon
Serves: 4

Ingredients
- 2 Sweet Potatoes, Sliced
- 4 Oz. Bacon, Cooked And Crumbled
- 1 C. Fresh Salsa
- 1 Tsp. Chili Powder
- ½ Tsp. Garlic Powder
- ½ Tsp. Paprika
- 2 Tbsp. Extra-Virgin Olive Oil
- Fresh Cilantro, Finely Chopped
- Salt And Pepper
- 2 Avocados, Chopped
- 1 Garlic Clove, Finely Chopped
- 1 Tbsp. Fresh Lime Juice
- ½ C. Roma Tomatoes, Chopped
- ¼ C. Red Onion, Chopped

Directions
1. Preheat the oven to 450 degrees.
2. Mash the avocados until they're smooth. Add all the rest of the ingredients for the guacamole and stir until combined. Cover and refrigerate.

3. Put the potatoes in the bowl and drizzle with oil. Sprinkle with paprika, chili powder, salt and pepper, and garlic powder. Toss until well coated.
4. Put the sweet potatoes in the baking sheet and cook for twelve minutes on either side.
5. Top with the potatoes with the salsa, guacamole, bacon bits, and cilantro.

Sausage-Stuffed Jalapeño Bites
Serves: 4

Ingredients
- 1 Lb. Italian Sausage, Casing Removed
- 1 Onion, Chopped
- ¼ C. Almond Flour
- 1 Egg Beaten
- 1 Lb. Jalapeño Peppers, Halved And Seeded
- ½ Tbsp. Dried Oregano
- Cooking Fat
- Salt And Pepper

Directions
1. Preheat the oven to 425 degrees.
2. Melt the fat in a skillet and brown the sausage for five minutes and let it cool.
3. Combine the onion, sausage meat, beaten egg, flour, oregano, and season to taste. Stir until combined.
4. Spoon a tablespoon of sausage over the jalapeno halves.
5. Put them on a baking sheet and bake in the oven for twenty minutes.

Creamy Garlic Mushrooms

Serves: 4

Ingredients

- 16 Oz. Mushrooms, Cleaned And Destemmed
- 4 Cloves Of Garlic, Finely Chopped
- ½ C. Coconut Cream
- 2 Tbsp. Clarified Butter
- 2 Fresh Thyme Sprigs
- 2 Tbsp. Olive Oil
- Salt And Pepper

Directions

1. Preheat the oven to 375 degrees.
2. Melt the fat in a skillet over medium heat.
3. Add the garlic and sauté for three minutes.
4. Add the thyme and cook another minute.
5. Put the mushrooms with the cap side down on top of the thyme and the garlic.
6. Season the mushrooms with salt and pepper to taste.
7. Drizzle with the oil and roast in the oven fifteen minutes.
8. Remove the skillet and put it on the stovetop over low heat.
9. Pour in the milk and keep cooking over low heat until warm. Scrape up the browned bits.
10. Remove the thyme and serve warm.

Roasted Butternut Squash And Turnips

Serves: 4

Ingredients

- 2 Small Turnips, Peeled And Chopped
- 1 Butternut Squash, Peeled And Chopped
- 1 C. Fresh Cranberries
- 1 C. Pecans, Coarsely Chopped
- 1 Tsp. Ground Cinnamon
- ¼ Tsp. Nutmeg
- ¼ Tsp. Allspice
- 2 Tbsp. Olive Oil
- Fresh Parsley, To Garnish

Directions

1. Preheat the oven to 400 degrees.
2. In a bowl, combine the turnip, squash, spices, and olive oil in a bowl. Season to taste.
3. Toss the turnips and squash until coated with the spices and oil.
4. Spread the vegetables on the greased baking sheet and put them in the oven. Bake half an hour.
5. Remove the baking sheet from the oven, add the pecan, and add the cranberries. Toss.
6. Return it to the oven and cook fifteen minutes.
7. Serve garnished with parsley.

Roasted Brussels Sprouts with Grapes
Serves: 4

Ingredients
- 4 C. Fresh Brussels Sprouts, Halved
- 2 C. Seedless Red Grapes
- 2 Tbsp. Fresh Thyme
- ½ C. Walnuts, Coarsely Chopped
- 2 Tbsp. Olive Oil
- 1 Tbsp. Balsamic Vinegar
- Salt And Pepper

Directions
1. Preheat the oven to 400 degrees.
2. Combine the grapes and Brussels sprouts in a bowl.
3. Drizzle with olive oil, thyme, vinegar, and season to taste.
4. Transfer to a baking sheet and roast for half an hour.
5. Garnish with the walnuts and roast ten minutes.
6. Serve warm.

Dill Potato Salad
Serves: 4

Ingredients

- 2 Lbs. Yukon Gold Potatoes, Peeled
- ¼ Red Onion, Finely Chopped
- 2 Celery Stalks, Finely Chopped
- 3 Tbsp. Fresh Dill, Chopped
- 3 Anchovy Filets, Finely Chopped
- ½ C. Homemade Mayonnaise
- 1 Tbsp. Lemon Juice
- 2 Tsp. Dijon Mustard
- ½ Tbsp. Apple Cider Vinegar
- Salt And Pepper

Directions

1. Put the potatoes in a pot and cover with water. Season to taste and bring to a boil.
2. Cook the potatoes twenty minutes or until tender.
3. Drain and cool.
4. Cube the potatoes.
5. Stir the mayonnaise, anchovy filets, lemon juice, Dijon mustard, and apple cider vinegar. Season to taste.
6. Add the celery, potatoes, dill, onion, and mix to combine.
7. Taste and adjust the seasoning.
8. Serve chilled.

Garlic Green Beans
Serves: 4

Ingredients

- 1 Lb. Green Beans, Trimmed
- 3 Cloves Of Garlic, Finely Chopped
- ¼ C. Coconut Aminos
- 2 Tbsp. Clarified Butter
- 1 Tbsp. Rice Vinegar
- ¼ Tsp. Sesame Oil, Optional
- Sea Salt To Taste

Directions

1. Bring a pot of water to a boil and season with salt over high heat.
2. Add the green beans and blanch two minutes.
3. Transfer to an ice bath to stop cooking and drain.
4. Heat the butter in a sauté pan over medium heat.
5. Once hot, add the garlic and sauté for half a second.
6. Add the coconut aminos, green beans, vinegar, rice, and sesame oil. Toss.
7. Season to taste.
8. Cook five minutes, until the sauce has reduced and the green beans are tender.
9. Transfer to a serving bowl and drizzle the sauce over the green beans.

Roasted Mushrooms With Thyme
Serves: 4

Ingredients
- 16 Oz. Cremini Mushrooms
- 4 Cloves Of Garlic, Finely Chopped
- 8 Fresh Thyme Sprigs
- Butter
- 2 Tbsp. Olive Oil
- Salt And Pepper

Directions
1. Preheat the oven to 375 degrees.
2. Add the butter, thyme, and garlic to the bottom of an ovenproof skillet.
3. Put the mushrooms with the cap side down on the thyme and garlic.
4. Season to taste with salt and pepper.
5. Drizzle with the oil and roast in the oven for twenty-five minutes.
6. Remove the skillet from the oven and baste the mushrooms. Serve.

Blueberry-Peach Salsa
Serves: 4

Ingredients
- 4 Peaches, Peeled And Chopped
- 8 Oz. Blueberries
- ½ C. Pomegranate Seeds
- 1 Garlic Clove, Finely Chopped
- 1 Red Onion, Finely Chopped
- 1 Jalapeño Pepper, Finely Chopped
- 2 Tbsp. Fresh Chives, Finely Chopped
- 2 Tbsp. Fresh Basil, Finely Chopped
- 3 Tbsp. Fresh Lime Juice
- ¼ C. Fresh Peach Juice
- Salt And Pepper

Directions
1. Combine the lime juice, garlic, peach juice, and salt and pepper to taste in a bowl.
2. Combine the rest of the ingredients in a bowl.
3. Pour the lime juice mix over the salsa and give it all a good stir. Refrigerate.

Sweet Potato Nachos

Serves: 4

Ingredients

- 2 Large Sweet Potatoes, Peeled And Sliced Into ¼-Inch Thick Slices
- ¼ C. Green Onions, Chopped
- ½ C. Bell Peppers, Chopped
- 1 Avocado, Chopped
- 2 Jalapeños, Sliced
- 1 Tsp. Garlic Powder
- 1 Tsp. Paprika
- 1 Tbsp. Olive Oil
- Fresh Cilantro, Finely Chopped
- Fresh Salsa
- Salt And Pepper

Directions

1. Preheat the oven to 425 degrees.
2. Combine the sweet potato slices with the paprika, oil, garlic powder, and season to taste with the salt and pepper.
3. Mix until well combined.
4. Put the sweet potatoes on the baking sheet and bake for forty minutes, turning once.
5. Remove from the oven and top with the green onions, bell pepper, and jalapenos.

6. Return the potato slices to the oven and broil ten minutes.
7. Serve with the salsa, avocado, and cilantro.

Drinks

Pink Grapefruit Lemonade
Serves: 4

Ingredients
- 1 ¼ C. Lemon Juice
- 1 ¼ C. Pink Grapefruit Juice
- ¼ C. Honey
- 1 ¾ C. Water
- Ice

Directions
1. In a saucepan, combine the water and honey over medium heat until the honey has fully dissolved.
2. Mix the lemon juice, honey water, and grapefruit juice in a pitcher and stir well.
3. Add the lemon or grapefruit slices to the pitcher. Fill the pitcher with ice.
4. Serve.

Peach And Raspberry Lemonade
Serves: 4

Ingredients
- 3 Peaches, Sliced
- 1 C. Lemon Juice
- 6 Oz. Raspberries
- 6 C. Cold Water
- 3 Tbsp. Raw Honey

Directions
1. Combine a cup of water and the peaches, raspberries, and honey in a saucepan over medium heat.
2. Let it all simmer for five minutes.
3. Pour the peach and raspberry mix in a blender until its smooth.
4. Strain the liquid through a mesh to remove the raspberry seeds.
5. Pour the mix into the pitcher and whisk in the lemon juice and the rest of the five cups of water.
6. Refrigerate and serve chilled with the ice.

Pomegranate Green Tea

Serves: 2

Ingredients

- 2 Tsp. Green Tea Leaves
- 2 Tsp. Pomegranate Seeds
- 6 Tbsp. Pomegranate Juice
- 1 ½ C. Boiling Water

Directions

1. Steep the tea in the warm water for four minutes.
2. Stir in the juice.
3. Pour the tea into two cups and add the seeds.

Watermelon Sport Drink

Serves: 1

Ingredients

- 1 C. Coconut Water
- Juice From Half A Lime
- 1 C. Watermelon, Cut Into Cubes
- Salt

Directions

1. Combine everything in a blender and pulse until smooth.

Coconut Milk Hot Chocolate

Serves: 2

Ingredients

- 13.5 oz. can full fat coconut milk
- ¼ tsp. vanilla extract
- 1.5 oz. dark chocolate, finely chopped

Directions

1. Heat the milk in a pan over medium heat until hot, but not boiling.
2. Add the vanilla and chocolate and stir until melted.
3. Serve hot.

Coconut Strawberry Lemonade

Serves: 2

Ingredients

- 6 Mint Leaves
- 2 Lime Slices
- 2 Lemon Slices
- 6 Strawberries, Sliced
- 2 C. Coconut Water
- 2 Tbsp. Fresh Lime Juice
- 2 Tbsp. Fresh Lemon Juice
- 1 Tbsp. Raw Honey

Directions

1. Mash the lemon, mint, and lime slices with a mortar and pestle.
2. Scoop the mash into a lemonade pitcher and add the lime and lemon juice.
3. Add all the rest of the ingredients and stir it. Chill and serve over ice.

Lemon Mint Iced Tea

Serves: 4-6

Ingredients

- 3 C. Of Good Quality Tea, Chilled
- 1 Lemon, Sliced
- 8 Fresh Mint Leaves
- 1 Lime, Sliced
- Ice Cubes

Directions

1. In a jar, put the lime and lemon slices, as well as the mint.
2. Fill the jar with the cubes and the tea and stir.
3. Chill in the refrigerator for four to six hours before serving.

Raspberry lime Flavored Water
Serves: 4

Ingredients
- 6 Oz. Of Raspberries
- Ice Cubes
- 2 Limes, Quartered
- Water

Directions
1. Squeeze the juice from the limes into your jar and toss in the lime quarters, too.
2. Add the raspberries and squeeze gently, making sure not to break them.
3. Add the ice to the jar and pour the water in until it's full. Stir it up and refrigerate.

Lemonade with Thyme

Serves: 1

Ingredients

- 3 Tbsp. Freshly Squeezed Lemon Juice
- A Few Ice Cubes
- 2 C. Cold Water
- 1 Sprig Fresh Thyme

Directions

1. Combine the water, lemon juice, and ice cubes. Stir and serve with the thyme sprig. Strain the lemon pulp before serving.

Strawberry Rhubarb Lemonade

Serves: 6

Ingredients

- 3 ½ C. Water
- 1 Lb. Rhubarb, Chopped
- 3 C. Fresh Strawberries, Halved
- Zest Of 2 Lemons
- 1 ½ C. Freshly Squeezed Lemon Juice

Directions

1. In a pot of water, combine the lemon zest and rhubarb. Let it come to a boil. Once boiling, reduce the heat and keep simmering for fifteen minutes. At this point, add the strawberries and cook three minutes.
2. Remove from the heat and let it cool completely. Once the mix is at room temperature. Use a hand blender to puree it. When a smooth texture takes form, stir in the lemon juice.
3. Put the lemonade in the refrigerator until it was cold before serving.

Desserts

Pumpkin Pie Pudding
Serves: 4

Ingredients

- ½ C. Canned Unsweetened Pumpkin Purée
- ¼ C. Raw Honey
- 1 ¾ C. Coconut Milk
- 2 Tbsp. Tapioca Starch
- 1 Tbsp. Water
- 1 Egg
- 1 Tsp. Pure Vanilla Extract
- ⅛ Tsp. Ground Allspice
- ¼ Tsp. Ground Nutmeg
- ½ Tsp Ground Cinnamon
- ¼ Tsp. Ground Ginger

Directions

1. In a bowl, combine the tapioca and water until the starch has dissolved.
2. In the saucepan, mix the coconut milk, honey, and egg together.
3. Bring the coconut milk mix to a boil as you whisk. Pour in the water mix as you continue to whisk.
4. Cook for two minutes and remove from the heat.

5. In a bowl, combine the pumpkin with the rest of the ingredient and whisk until blended.
6. Slowly add the pumpkin puree mix to the coconut milk and whisk constantly, putting it over low heat.
7. Cook for three to four minutes.
8. Divide the pudding amongst dessert bowls and chill until it's set, one to two hours.

Fruit Banana Split
Serves: 2

Ingredients

- ¼ C. Nuts Of Your Choice, Roasted And Chopped
- 2 Bananas, Peeled And Sliced Lengthwise
- Fresh Fruits, Sliced
- ½ C. Fresh Strawberries, Sliced
- ½ C. Fresh Blueberries
- ¼ C. Raw Honey
- ▯ C. Water

Directions

1. Combine the water and honey in a saucepan over medium heat.
2. Stir in the strawberries and blueberries and stir until well mixed.
3. Bring it to a boil and lower the heat and simmer five minutes.
4. Pour the sauce into the food processor and pulse until smooth.
5. Arrange the banana on a plate and top with the fresh fruits of your choice.
6. Drizzle the strawberry and blueberry sauce over the banana and sprinkle with the roasted nuts.

Coconut Date Balls

Serves: 4

Ingredients

- 1 C. Dates, Roughly Chopped
- 2 Eggs, Beaten
- ½ C. Raw Honey
- 1 Tsp. Vanilla Extract
- ¼ C. Ghee
- 2 C. Mixed Nuts, Chopped Small
- 1 C. Coconut Flakes
- ½ Tsp. Sea Salt

Directions

1. Combine the butter with the eggs, honey, and dates in a saucepan over medium heat.
2. Bring it to a boil and stir for three to five minutes.
3. Remove it from the heat and stir in the vanilla and salt.
4. Mix in the nuts and stir until combined.
5. Roll the mix into balls.
6. Roll every ball in the flakes until it's well covered.
7. Refrigerate until it's firm.

Pumpkin Pie Bites
Serves: 4

Ingredients

- 1 ½ C. Pumpkin Puree
- 2 Ripe Bananas
- 1 Egg
- ¼ C. Honey
- ¼ Tsp. Ground Ginger
- 1 Tsp. Ground Cinnamon
- ¼ Tsp. Ground Nutmeg
- ¼ Tsp. Salt
- 1 Can Full Fat Coconut Milk
- 2 Egg Whites
- 1 Tsp. Pure Vanilla Extract

Directions

1. Preheat the oven to 350 degrees.
2. Combine the pumpkin through the coconut milk together in a bowl and blend until smooth.
3. Spoon into muffin cups.
4. Bake in the oven for half an hour.
5. In a bowl, whip the egg whites until they make white peaks. Add the coconut milk as you blend.
6. Keep blending until you get a creamy texture and add in the vanilla.

7. Top the bites with the whipped cream and serve.

Chocolate Dipped Apples
Serves: 6

Ingredients
- 6 Apples
- 1 Lb. Of White Chocolate, Chunked
- 1 C. Of Each Topping Choice, Chopped Nuts
- 6 Popsicle Sticks

Directions
1. Wash the apples and twist off the stems. Push a stick into the core of every apple.
2. The chocolate adheres to the apples if they're cold, so put the apples in the refrigerator as you prepare everything else.
3. Put your topping choices in the bowls. It's best to be sure the toppings are small pieces because nothing too big will stick.
4. Heat the chocolate in the double boiler or in the microwave until it's fully melted. Remove it from the heat and stir it until fully melted and warm.
5. Dip the apples in the chocolate and pull them up to let the chocolate drip off.
6. Put on a waxed paper lined baking sheet and refrigerate until the chocolate has set, around half an hour.

Strawberry Applesauce
Serves: 4

Ingredients
- 12 Large Strawberries, Chopped
- 4 Lb. Apples, Peeled, Cored, And Chopped
- ¼ C. Raw Honey
- Juice From ½ Lemon
- ¼ Tsp. Pure Vanilla Extract
- ¼ Tsp. Ground Allspice

Directions
1. Combine everything in a saucepan.
2. Set the heat to medium and bring it to a simmer for forty-five minutes.
3. Use an emulsion blender to pulse and break up any lumps to make a smooth sauce.

Chocolate Oranges
Serves: 4

Ingredients
- 5 Mandarin Oranges, Peeled
- ½ C. Dark Chocolate
- Sea Salt

Directions
1. Line a baking sheet with some parchment paper.
2. Melt the chocolate with a double boiler over boiling water on medium-low heat.
3. Dip the orange slice halfway into the chocolate and put it on the baking sheet.
4. Garnish with chocolate covered orange slices with salt.
5. Refrigerate for ten minutes and serve.

Banana Ice Cream

Serves: 2-3

Ingredients

- 3 Ripe Bananas
- Coconut Flakes
- Dark Chocolate, Shaved
- Orange Zest
- Chopped Nuts

Directions

1. Begin by peeling the bananas and slicing them.
2. Put the slices in a bowl and process until smooth. This process takes a while and you have to scrape down the sides of the food processor with a spatula.
3. The bananas will crumble and you will end up with a soft mix.
4. At this point, put it back in the glass bowl and freeze for an hour.
5. Garnish with toppings.

Almond and Coconut Macaroons
Serves: 4

Ingredients
- 2 Egg Whites
- 2 C. Unsweetened Shredded Coconut
- ¼ C. Raw Honey
- ½ C. Whole Almonds, Chopped Into Tiny Pieces
- 1 Tsp. Pure Vanilla Extract

Directions
1. Preheat the oven to 350 degrees.
2. Line a baking pan with parchment paper.
3. In a bowl, whisk the egg whites and honey together.
4. Add the shredded coconut, almonds, and vanilla to the bowl and mix.
5. Form the dough into macaroons. Drop onto the prepared sheet and put it in the oven.
6. Bake until the bottoms are golden, twelve minutes.

Fried Honey Banana

Serves: 1

Ingredients

- 1 Banana, Sliced
- Cinnamon
- 1 Tbsp. Honey
- 2 Tbsp. Coconut Oil

Directions

1. Combine the honey with a quarter of a cup of water and mix it well.
2. Heat the oil in a skillet over medium heat.
3. Add the banana slices and fry for two minutes on either side.
4. Remove the skillet from the hat and pour the honey over the top.
5. Sprinkle with cinnamon.

Snacks

Baked Apple Chips
Serves: 4

Ingredients
- 3 Apples
- Ground Cinnamon, To Taste

Directions
1. Preheat the oven to 220 degrees.
2. Line the baking sheet with parchment paper and set it aside.
3. Cut the apples into thin slices.
4. Spread the apple slices on the baking sheet, making sure you have no overlapping edges.
5. Sprinkle with cinnamon and put it in the oven.
6. Put them in the oven and dry for an hour and then flip the slices and cook for an hour.
7. Let the chips cool and serve.

Pineapple with Lime and Mint
Serves: 4

Ingredients
- 1 Fresh Pineapple
- Fresh Mint Leaves, Finely Chopped
- Zest And Juice Of 1 Lime

Directions
1. Slice the top and bottom off the pineapple and stand it up. Slice the sides off.
2. Cut it into four thick slices.
3. Sprinkle with the lime zest, juice, and finely chopped mint over the pineapple and serve.

Apple and Almond Butter Bites
Serves: 2

Ingredients
- 1 Apple, Cored And Thinly Sliced
- Pecans, Chopped
- Almond Butter
- Almonds, Sliced
- Dark Chocolate Chips
- Roasted Coconut Shreds
- Dried Cranberries

Directions
1. Spread the almond butter over a side of the apple slice.
2. Top the slices with your choices of toppings.

Raspberry-Lime Fruit Dip
Serves: 4

Ingredients
- 1 C. Raspberries, Drained
- 2 Tbsp. Lime Juice
- 1 C. Full-Fat Coconut Milk
- 1 Tsp. Lime Peel, Grated
- 2 Tbsp. Honey

Directions
1. Put the raspberries in the blender and pulse until it's smooth.
2. Strain the puree and discard the seeds.
3. Combine the honey, coconut milk, lime zest, lime juice, and raspberry sauce together. Stir until well blended.
4. Serve cold with some fresh fruits.

Honey-Coated Walnuts and Peaches
Serves: 4

Ingredients
- 4 Peaches, Quartered
- ¼ C. Raw Honey
- ½ C. Walnuts, Chunked
- ¼ C. Clarified Butter
- 1 Tsp. Ground Cinnamon

Directions
1. Melt the butter in a skillet and the honey for two to three minutes.
2. Add the cinnamon and peaches to the mix and cook for five minutes.
3. Add the walnuts and cook for another three minutes.
4. Serve with a scoop of ice cream.

Fruit Pudding
Serves: 4

Ingredients
- 1 Lb. Frozen Fruit
- 2 C. Of Orange Juice
- 5 Tbsp. Tapioca Starch
- 4 Fresh Mint Leaves

Directions
1. Bring the fruit and orange juice to a simmer in a pan over medium heat and simmer a few minutes. Strain through a sieve into a bowl.
2. Put the fruit in the sieve in another bowl and refrigerate.
3. Pour the strained fruit back into the saucepan and bring it to a simmer.
4. As the mix simmers, combine the starch with the water and some of the fruit juice in a bowl. Add the saucepan, stirring it until the mix thickens.
5. Pour the mix into four serving glasses, and chill for two hours or overnight.
6. Serve with a splash of the cooked fruits and mint leaf.

Chunky Fruit Popsicles
Serves: 8-10

Ingredients
- 1 Lb. Of Your Favorite Fruits
- Juice From 1 Orange
- Juice Of 1 Lemon
- ½ C. Of Water
- ¼ Tsp. Vanilla Extract

Directions
1. Cut a cup of the fruit into small chunks and set it aside.
2. Use a food processor to puree the rest of the fruits, lemon juice, orange juice, and the water until it's smooth.
3. Add the mix to the bowl with the chunky fruit and stir in the vanilla extract.
4. Divide the mix amongst the Popsicle molds.
5. Freeze for three to four hours.

Apple Cinnamon Fruit Rolls
Serves: 4

Ingredients
- 8 C. Of Apple, Peeled And Chopped
- 1 C. Water
- 1 Tbsp. Ground Cinnamon
- 2 Tbsp. Freshly Squeezed Lemon Juice

Directions
1. Put the apples in a saucepan over medium heat. Add the water and cover it. Let it simmer for fifteen minutes. Stir a few times to make sure it cooks consistently.
2. Put the apples into a food processor and pulse until smooth.
3. Pour the ingredients into the pot over a medium low temperature. Add the cinnamon and lemon juice. Continue cooking for ten more minutes.
4. Spoon the mix onto dehydrate trays. Be sure to keep the mix as level as possible as it dehydrates. Dehydrate at 135 degree for eight to twelve hours.
5. Cut the fruit leather into shaped rectangles and roll it to make fruit rolls.

Grilled Peaches With Prosciutto And Basil

Serves: 4

Ingredients

- 8 Slices Good Quality Prosciutto
- 3 Ripe Peaches, Halved And Pitted
- 1 C. Balsamic Vinegar
- 1 Tbsp. Honey, Optional
- 10 Basil Leaves
- 2 Tbsp. Coconut Oil, Melted
- Salt And Pepper To Taste

Directions

1. In a saucepan over medium heat, bring the vinegar to a simmer for a few minutes. As it thickens, add the honey, and season to taste. Once it looks like thick syrup, remove it from the heat and let it cool.
2. Heat your grill to medium heat and brush some of the oil over the open sides of the peaches. Put them on the grill face down and let them cook until golden. Cook on the other side for another minute.
3. Put the peaches face up on a flat dish and drizzle with the vinegar syrup and stuff the pit with prosciutto. Garnish with basil and serve.

Homemade Yogurt

Serves: 4

Ingredients

- 4 C. Whole Milk
- Powder Bacterial Starter

Directions

1. Pour the milk into a pan and heat it over medium low. Bring it to 180 degrees.
2. Cool the milk to room temperature.
3. Add the powder starter according to its directions.
4. Pour into a glass jar and cover with plastic wrap. Put it in the oven with your light on.
5. Let it ferment for twenty-four hours.
6. Put the jar in the refrigerator, cool, and enjoy with fresh fruits!

Sauces and Dips

Sweet Potato Hummus
Serves: 4

Ingredients
- 4 C. Cooked And Mashed Sweet Potatoes
- ¼ C. Tahini (Directions Below)
- ¼ C. Lime Juice
- 2 Cloves Of Garlic, Finely Chopped
- ¼ Tsp. Cayenne Pepper
- 2 Tsp. Ground Cumin
- Salt And Pepper
- 1 C. Sesame Seeds:
- 2 Tbsp. Olive Oil

Directions
1. Cook the sweet potatoes and peel them off. Cut the flesh into chunks. Bring a pot of water with salt to boil and add in the sweet potato chunks.
2. Allow it to simmer for ten minutes until the flesh is tender.
3. Drain, put the cooked sweet potato in a bowl and mash with a fork. Put in the refrigerator to cool.
4. Preheat the oven to 350 degrees.
5. Spread the seeds on a baking tray and roast, shaking until fragrant.

6. Prepare the tahini and combine the toasted sesame seeds with the oil in a food processor. Process until it's smooth, around five minutes.
7. In a bowl, combine the sweet potatoes, lime juice, tahini, cumin, garlic, and cayenne.
8. Mix everything and season to taste.

Sriracha Sauce
Serves: 3-4

Ingredients
- 1½ Lbs. Red Hot Peppers, Chopped
- 4 Thai Chilies, Sliced
- 5 Cloves Of Garlic
- 3 Tbsp. White Wine Vinegar
- 2 Tbsp. Raw Honey
- 2 Tbsp. Tomato Paste
- 2 Tbsp. Fish Sauce
- 2 Tbsp. Extra-Virgin Olive Oil
- Sea Salt, To Taste

Directions
1. Put the red peppers, chilies, and garlic in a food processor.
2. Add the rest of the ingredients and pulse until smooth.
3. Season to taste. If the sauce is too thick, add a tablespoon of water.
4. Pour the sauce into a pan and bring it to a boil over medium heat.
5. Reduce the heat to low and let it simmer ten minutes.
6. Let the sauce cool down and pour it into a jar.

Red Pepper Dip

Serves: 8-10

Ingredients

- 2 C. Pecans, Almonds, Macadamia Nuts Or Walnuts
- ½ Tsp. Ground Cumin
- 2 Tbsp. Homemade Mayonnaise
- 2 Tbsp. Extra Virgin Olive Oil
- 12 Oz. Jar Roasted Red Peppers, Drained
- 2 Tbsp. Fresh Lemon Juice
- Salt And Pepper To Taste

Directions

1. Put the nuts in a food processor and pulse until they're crumbs. Add the cumin, mayonnaise, and salt and pepper and keep mixing until it's evenly combined.
2. Add the rest of the ingredients in the food processor and process until it takes the form and consistency of dip.
3. Taste and add salt and pepper, and lemon juice, if desired.

Coconut Paleo Mayonnaise
Serves: 1.25 Cups

Ingredients
- 2 Egg Yolks
- 3 Tsp. Lemon Juice
- 1 Tsp. Mustard
- ½ C. Olive Oil
- ½ C. Coconut Oil

Directions
1. In a bowl, mix the mustard, yolks, and a teaspoon of lemon juice.
2. Start whisking or put a food processor on low.
3. Emulsify slowly with the oil and enjoy.

Paleo Baba-Ghanoush
Serves: 8

Ingredients
- 2 Large Eggplants
- 2 Cloves Of Garlic, Finely Chopped
- 2 Tbsp. Tahini
- 2 Tbsp. Fresh Lemon Juice
- 3 Tsp. Extra-Virgin Olive Oil
- 1 Tsp. Cumin
- Salt And Pepper To Taste
- Fresh Parsley, Garnishing

Directions
1. Roast the eggplants on a grill. Darken the skin evenly. Prick the skin with a fork and roast thirty-five minutes in the oven at 400 degrees.
2. Put the roasted eggplants in a bowl of cold water and then peel off the skin.
3. Put the roasted eggplant, lemon juice, garlic, olive oil, tahini, and cumin in a blender and pulse until smooth. Season to taste.
4. Cool in the refrigerator and serve with parsley as a garnish.

Quick and Easy Guacamole
Serves: 2.5 Cups

Ingredients
- 3 Avocados
- 1 Tomato, Finely Chopped
- ½ White Onion
- ½ C. Chopped Cilantro
- 2 Tbsp. Fresh Lemon Juice
- Salt And Pepper

Directions
1. Scoop out the avocado flesh. Mash the flesh with a fork.
2. Stir the other ingredients in.
3. Enjoy or store it in the refrigerator right away.

Salsa Verde

Serves: 4

Ingredients

- ½ C. Onion, Chopped
- 1 ½ Lbs. Green Tomatillos, Husk Removed
- ½ C. Cilantro, Chopped
- 2 Tbsp. Lime Juice
- 2 Jalapeño Peppers, Seeded And Chopped
- Salt And Pepper

Directions

1. Cut the tomatillos in half and roast them on the grill for six minutes under the broiler.
2. Put the roasted tomatillos, cilantro, onion, jalapeno, and lime juice in a food processor.
3. Pulse until blended.
4. Cool in the fridge and enjoy.

Homemade Basil Pesto
Serves: 1 Cup

Ingredients
- 2 Packed C. Fresh Basil Leaves
- ½ C. Good Quality Extra Virgin Olive Oil
- ½ C. Parmesan Cheese
- ⬚ C. Pine Nuts
- 3 Cloves Of Garlic, Finely Chopped
- Salt And Pepper

Directions
1. Put the garlic, basil, and nuts in a food processor and pulse until it's chopped.
2. Add the oil and parmesan and pulse again until smooth.
3. Season to taste.
4. Enjoy or freeze.

Strawberry Balsamic Vinaigrette
Serves: 4

Ingredients
- 1 C. Strawberries
- ¼ C. Balsamic Vinegar
- ¼ C. Extra-Virgin Olive Oil
- 1 Tbsp. Dijon Mustard
- 1 Clove Garlic, Finely Chopped
- ¼ Tsp. Salt
- ¼ Tsp. Pepper

Directions
1. Preheat the oven to 425 degrees.
2. Rinse the strawberries, remove the stems, and line a baking sheet with foil. Fold the edges up to make a well on all sides to prevent juices from coming out. Roast for twenty minutes.
3. Add everything to a blender and be sure to include the juices that came out of the berries. Puree the mix until smooth and consistent. Serve cold and refrigerate.

Sardine And Garlic Spread
Serves: 4-6

Ingredients
- 1 Head Of Garlic
- 8 Sardine Fillets
- 2 Tbsp. Capers
- 12 Tbsp. Extra-Virgin Olive Oil
- 2 Tbsp. Red Wine Vinegar
- Olive Oil
- Salt And Pepper

Directions
1. Preheat the oven to 400 degrees.
2. Peel away the outer layers of skin, but avoid pulling off too much.
3. Cut off the top of the bulb.
4. Put the bulb on foil and drizzle the oil. Sprinkle with salt and pepper.
5. Gather the ends and close the bulb in. put the foiled garlic on the baking sheet and bake half an hour.
6. Pull open the foil so the heat escapes and the bulbs. Once they've cooled, pop out the cloves.
7. Put the garlic, capers, sardines, and vinegar into a blende rand pulse until a smooth paste forms.
8. Taste and season.
9. Keep blending and slowly pour in the oil.

10. Serve or refrigerate for later.

Conclusion

Thank you again for purchasing this book!

I hope this book was able to help you to learn how to cook delicious Paleo recipes.

The next step is to create a menu plan and get started with cooking.

Finally, if you enjoyed this book, then I'd like to ask you for a favor, would you be kind enough to leave a review for this book on Amazon? It'd be greatly appreciated!

Thank you and good luck!

Made in the USA
Lexington, KY
11 June 2016